"I am a forty-four-year-old pediatric physical therapist and I was given your book by one of my clients. It is fantastic! After doing the program for one week I went out and bought six more books to give as gifts for Christmas and have recommended it to countless other women! My forty-one-year-old sister is seven months pregnant and asked her OB about starting the program, and her OB wants to recommend it to every woman in her clinic! I have been doing the program now for six weeks, today just started the third level, and I now feel ten years younger."

—*Terry Geisberger*

"I am fifteen and in high school. I have gradually worked my way up to the Ultimate Core and have seen myself get more flexible and toned. I have recommended this program to my mom (age fifty), sister (age twelve), grandma (age eighty-one), and several of my friends and they have gotten excellent results too!"

—*A reader from Glenview, Illinois, on Amazon*

"I'm not very flexible and am constantly lifting my sixteen-month-old daughter. Needless to say, my back is continually aching. Even though I've only been doing this program for a week, already the soreness is diminished to the point where it is almost gone. I really thought I would have to deal with back pain for the rest of my life. What a relief, in more ways than one, to know I can do something about it. As an added bonus, my stomach is getting flatter—something that hasn't happened since before I was pregnant!"

—*A reader from Pittsburgh, on Amazon*

"I've only been doing Peggy's exercises for six weeks, but the results I've seen—and my chiropractor has seen—are thrilling! Before I started, I was seeing my chiropractor twice a week for my lower-back problems. After a short time, I dropped to once a week. As of my last visit, my back was holding up so well that he said I could drop to once every two weeks. This is an amazing progression in only six weeks!

"I feel strong, and the body fat around my waist, thighs, and hips seems to be melting away. I was sore at first, but in a short time I am doing exercises well that I originally rolled my eyes at when I started. The book is easy to understand and follow because at the end of each section, she has a two-page pictorial review of all the exercises in that section.

"If everyone got this book, a lot of health practitioners would be out of business."

—*Artie Dewey, on Amazon*

"I am forty-six years old, married with two children, and I work full-time (most of it sitting behind a computer). I have struggled with stress-related neck and back problems for the last five years and recently found out that I also have arthritis in my neck. Recently I had hit a new low in that I was having migraine-level headaches and nausea, in addition to constant muscle spasms and facial and arm tingling. However, when I started doing the Core Foundation exercises, I eliminated the headaches and muscle spasms and was also able to use the exercises during the day to relieve muscle tension. The fact that the program a) takes fifteen minutes once a day, b) doesn't involve going to lessons or a gym, and c) that I immediately felt better seemed too good to be true—but it is!!!"

—*Barbara Colling*

"I had back surgery earlier this year and had resigned myself to living with a certain amount of pain. This book really changed that. After following the program for three weeks, I feel better than ever. I'm sleeping better, have no pain, am standing taller and walking straighter. I have recommended this book to every woman I know. It is written in easy-to-understand language and the exercises are easy to follow. And there are no sit-ups!!!"

—*Monica O'Neal, on Amazon*

"I never thought I'd be free from back pain due to arthritis and hard living for my first forty years. Now forty-nine, I started the Core Program three and a half weeks ago and have just had four days in a row with absolutely NO PAIN! I'm ecstatic. I'm starting to believe my second forty years will be enjoyable after all!"

—*Kathy Okay*

"When I first got this book, I had high hopes. . . . The first time I did the workout, however, I was slightly disappointed and thought maybe this isn't for me. Then an amazing thing happened. The next day, after just one workout session, I actually felt a difference! Now I am a believer and recommend this book to everyone. The reason I was mildly disappointed the first time doing the exercises is that they are so easy, I felt like I wasn't 'doing' anything. That is one of the great things about this program—it is very relaxing, with a lot of gentle stretching and just a few strength-building exercises; it is not rigorous, traditional exercise, so there is no excuse not to do it as part of your daily routine. In fact, I think you will look forward to your core exercise time.

"Aside from the exercises, the author gives a lot of information about how the body functions, proper postures when sitting, sleeping, and lifting objects, and lots of other really useful info. This book is a MUST have."

—*A reader from Virginia, on Amazon*

the**core**program

FIFTEEN MINUTES A DAY
THAT CAN CHANGE YOUR LIFE

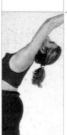

BY PEGGY W. BRILL, P.T.
with GERALD S. COUZENS
Photos by MARC WITZ

BANTAM BOOKS
NEW YORK TORONTO LONDON SYDNEY AUCKLAND

This edition contains the complete text
of the original hardcover edition.
NOT ONE WORD HAS BEEN OMITTED.

THE CORE PROGRAM

A Bantam Book

PUBLISHING HISTORY

Bantam hardcover edition published September 2001.
Bantam trade paperback edition / January 2003

The exercises and suggestions in this book are guidelines for the healthy individual. If you have specific medical problems or are unsure whether you should perform certain exercises, please consult your physician or physical therapist.

Library of Congress Catalog Card Number: 2001035258.

ISBN 0-553-38084-2

Published simultaneously in the United States and Canada

Bantam Books are published by Bantam Books, a division of Random House, Inc. Its trademark, consisting of the words "Bantam Books" and the portrayal of a rooster, is Registered in U.S. Patent and Trademark Office and in other countries. Marca Registrada. Bantam Books, New York, New York.

PRINTED IN THE UNITED STATES OF AMERICA

RRC   10   9   8   7   6   5

For my mother, whose love, affection and courage gave me strength to find my passion and to dream of leaving this world a better place

acknowledgments

I would like to express my deepest appreciation for the many people who've helped to make *The Core Program* possible. Some have contributed their efforts just recently, and others have blessed my life all along the way, influencing my emotional, mental, physical and spiritual evolution.

First and foremost, I must thank the patients who entrusted me with their health. They shared their physical and emotional pain with me, helping me to understand the power of the human spirit and the body's innate capacity to heal. My work as a physical therapist is as rewarding as it is because of my patients, who make each day so joyful for me.

One patient I would particularly like to thank is John J. Mack, who first came to me for an orthopedic problem and, in time, became my hero. John is the reason I was able to expand my practice at Morgan Stanley, and his incredible leadership inspires me. I am most fortunate for his mentoring and for the loving friendship I have with John and his beautiful wife, Christy. Thank you for all the doors you have so graciously and generously opened in my life.

I've also had the good fortune to have patients sent to me by Dr. Charles B. Goodwin, one of the best surgeons I have ever encountered. The success of my patients' rehabilitation was made possible by his amazing expertise and skills. Thank you for making my job a pleasure and thank you for welcoming me into the operating room, where I observed your outstanding work.

Gerald S. Couzens, my co-author, recognized the potential of my ideas and put them to paper so eloquently. Herb and Nancy Katz, my agents, had faith in my potential, saw the vision and went the extra mile for every part of it. Susan Suffes contributed her writing skills, and spent long hours translating medical explanations into reader-friendly terms with inspiring creativity.

My thanks to all those at Bantam who contributed to this project, especially my editors. I arrived with the hope that my book would be able to empower women with lifelong strength and health. Toni Burbank first directed that vision, and Beth Rashbaum clarified it with precision, expertise and meticulous detail.

I also thank Irwyn Applebaum, Bantam's publisher, for his brilliant title; Nita Taublib, deputy publisher, for her commitment to this project; Glen Edelstein and Kelly Chian in the production department for overseeing such a complicated process with such patience; Margaret Benton for the meticulous copyediting; Amanda Kavanagh for the elegant, energetic design of this book; and Marc Witz, who made the photo sessions playful as well as professional.

The work I do owes much to Margabandhu, my healer, who guided my recovery and restored my health, which inspired me to commit my life to the healing of others; and to Robin McKenzie, whose exceptional methodology for evaluating and treating disorders of the spine has been invaluable.

For love of my Scottish clan and pride in my roots, I extend my appreciation to all my cousins, aunts, uncles, and especially my beloved Grammie, whose unconditional love made me feel special. I thank my siblings—Lynette, Gregg and Russell—for their kindness and caring; they shaped my life more than they could ever imagine.

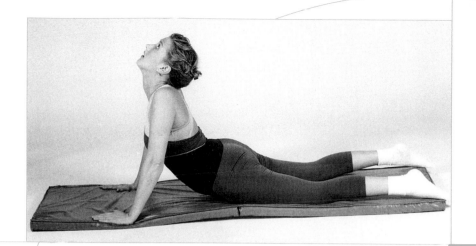

I thank my treasured friends Maria Hoelderlin, Tamar Amitay, Fern and Neil Zee, Stephanie Bologa, Melanie Fink, Christine Aragon, Elaine Stillerman and Roz Barrow Callahan for all their support and encouragement.

I thank my devoted staff for always striving to do their best: Gina Rosselli, Helen Corbet, Monica Joshi, Edward Broughton, Michael Ingino, Raymond Masselli, Vivian Andujar.

To my parents, Margaret and Alvin, whom I cherish—I give thanks every day for the life, love and support they gave me and the lessons they taught me. I would also like to thank my stepfather, Alfred Matthews, who brought me sunshine and comfort in some of my darkest moments. This book is dedicated to my adored mother, Margaret Bain-Matthews, who died three years ago at the age of 64 from a massive heart attack. My mother was beautiful, smart, funny, strong, affectionate and loving. I miss her every day and am grateful for all her blessings, especially her inspiration. Her loss was what motivated my crusade to protect other women from suffering—and this book is only the beginning.

My most profound appreciation goes to my husband, Gary, for his unrelenting dedication, and to our two beautiful, spirited little girls, Madison and Maggie—who are my life!

contents

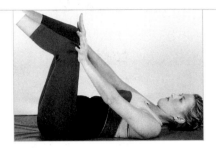

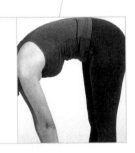

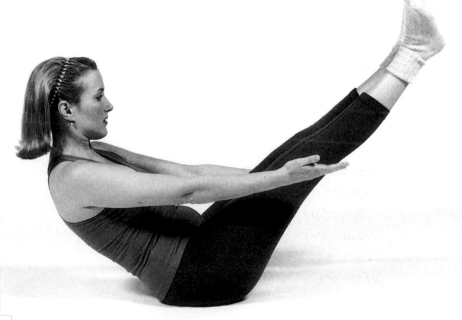

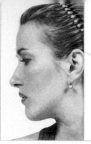

CONTENTS

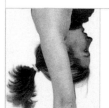

Charles B. Goodwin, M.D.

I tend to think of the work I do as a starting point in the restorative process, for it is only occasionally that I am able to treat a patient or complete a surgery without the need for follow-up care. More often than not, it is the physical therapy aftercare she receives, as well as her own determined effort to continue that therapy at home, that helps produce a truly successful outcome for my patient.

As a busy orthopedist, I have been privileged to work with many physical therapists over the years. All have labored long and hard to return my patients to good health by retraining and restoring strength and mobility to an injured muscle or limb, or by assisting them following surgery with special exercises and therapies. Clearly, some have been more successful than others at this very important work: Some do the job well; some shine; a few consistently set new standards along the way. I'm very happy to have made the acquaintance of one such rare bird—Peggy Brill—and so are my patients.

I now have the pleasure of working with Peggy as an integral part of my rehabilitation team. I find her powers of observation to be unusual, her compassion huge and her talent for healing quite extraordinary. Peggy has a unique appreciation for the workings of the human body and takes a holistic approach to body repair, a concept that I know to be an essential aspect of twenty-first-century medicine. For example, instead of providing therapy and exercises aimed only at strengthening an injured knee or lower back, Peggy actively encourages the patient to focus on developing and enhancing what she calls the "core" muscles. There's a powerful reason for this.

The core muscles are the large muscle groups of the back, abdomen, hips and pelvis. This is where strength and mobility originate. It's these important muscles that stabilize us as we move,

foreword

keeping the musculoskeletal (muscle and bone) structure in its proper place and in balance. A strong, mobile torso also equips us to handle the routine physical demands of daily life—carrying groceries, turning our head, neck and shoulder while backing out of a parking space, lifting children or simply getting up out of a chair—with more ease and fewer aches and pains.

The core work that Peggy recommends doesn't mean overbuilding these muscles; it means stretching and toning them, training them to work smoothly in concert with each other. By strengthening the muscles in your anatomic center—working this part of the body with great precision—you ultimately help prevent many musculoskeletal problems from developing. And by following Peggy's directions to concentrate on your breathing as you do your workout, you maximize the effectiveness of these exercises. Breathing deeply and evenly as you stretch your body will also enable you to release tension and relieve pent-up stress.

The Core Program is for everyone who wants to enjoy optimum health over the course of a lifetime. However, it may prove especially valuable to women over the age of 25, who are beginning to notice the tightening of tendons and muscles surrounding their joints. Although we all begin to see a natural loss of flexibility in supporting tissues around this time of life (much like the loss of elasticity that occurs in aging skin), more often than not these subtle changes become much more pronounced as our jobs and our family life become increasingly demanding, leaving us little time for physical activity. The net result of this progressive inactivity is that many routine physical movements formerly performed with great ease are now minefields of potential aches, pains and, yes, injuries.

To counter this, *The Core Program* gives you the information you need to develop a proactive strategy for taking care of your body, and doing it in just fifteen minutes a day. The core exercises help undo the muscle tightening and weakening that lead to pain and injury, thereby reversing any long-standing mechanical problems and preventing new ones.

As Peggy points out in *The Core Program*, your posture, your gait and even your breathing are all intimately related to your core muscles. By performing the exercises she recommends, you are working those muscles in a way that mimics the actual movements and functions you perform in real life, thus strengthening the body and preventing damage. This is a program that makes good sense for anyone, at any age and any level of fitness.

Just imagine yourself walking to work. With each step, the muscles of your hips, pelvis, abdomen and back contract to absorb the force of each footfall. But if the muscles of your back are weak, you may distort the way your foot lands, which not only leads to eventual problems with your foot, but in time to problems with your knee, hip and shoulder. Strengthening the core muscles, Peggy says, will keep this from occurring.

In addition to being a healer, Peggy is also a teacher. What you will come to like about *The Core Program* is that as you do the exercises you will learn how the various body parts work in symphony, how a stronger core enables you to move with greater ease and comfort and how to use these exercises to overcome injury and avoid recurrence.

Peggy addresses a variety of important subjects in *The Core Program*, including posture (the way you stand, sit and lie down), basic movement (how you walk and run) and your overall body mechanics (the way you use your body to perform everyday activities). *The Core Program* also provides advice to help you develop the flexibility your body needs. Many of my patients have commented that their bodies seem unusually agile and pain-free after just a few sessions of core exercises, especially when lifting heavy objects.

Look at *The Core Program* as a fitness guide and an exercise book rolled into one. Peggy's message is basic: Follow the easy-to-do preventive exercises outlined in her three specific programs and you will be doing all that you can do to protect the body's muscles, bones and ligaments. This prepares you to face the challenges of everyday life, including the demands of the workplace and any sports and exercise activities you choose.

The greatest secret weapon in this book is Peggy herself and her desire to share her healing arts with all of us. Her enthusiasm, commitment to health, and knowledge of physiology, anatomy and movement science are unique. I know you will find *The Core Program*, as I did, a truly exceptional offering.

what my core program will do for you

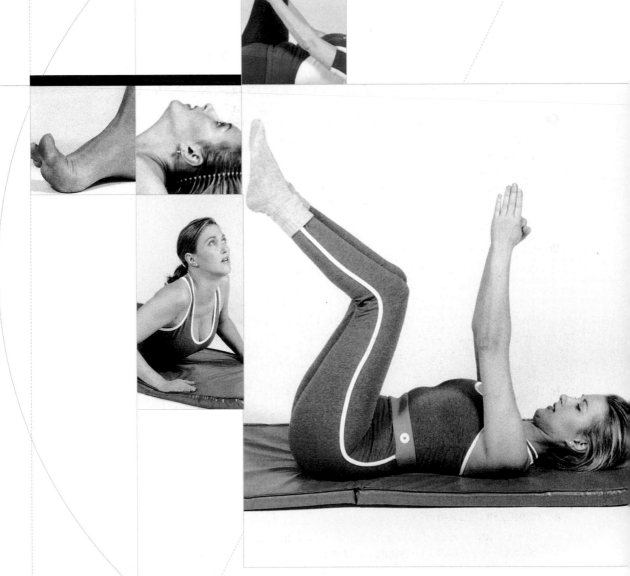

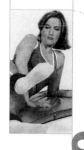

what every woman needs to know

chapter one

Can you imagine having all the energy you need, all the time?

Nancy, 32, has it. "Sitting at the computer all day used to leave me feeling drained. But now that I'm doing the core exercises, I don't feel like I've been run over by a truck by the end of the day. After work I'm taking a course in art school instead of dragging myself home and collapsing on the sofa."

Would you love to feel great every day?

Maria, 42, does. "For the first time in much too long I feel terrific, from head to toe. I never thought I'd feel this way again. I was dragging myself around, always feeling as if I were just one step away from moving at the pace of my 85-year-old grandmother. Best of all, I can accomplish everything I need to do, from lifting and carrying to walking long distances. I can't thank you enough!"

Is the notion of moving with ease and beautiful posture something you dream about?

For Jenna, 47, it is a reality. "Finally, I feel graceful; my strides are fluid. When I catch a glimpse of myself in a store window I see a confident woman, not someone who looks like she carries the weight of the world on her shoulders."

Do you wonder what it would be like to be able to summon strength anytime you needed it?

Carol, 36, can. "My arms and shoulders and even my hands were losing so much strength that I could barely carry my groceries. I figured it was just a sign of getting older. Not only do I really appreciate being proved wrong— now I don't have to think about whether I have the strength I need. It's always there."

Would you like to rid yourself of aches and pains once and for all?

> *Leslie, 40, did it. "Whenever I played on my company's soft-ball team I felt it the next day. Back strain. Shoulder pain. Now I'm a star hitter and the day after a game I can savor the victory—not try to soothe aches and pains."*

Is the idea of having dependable stamina immensely appealing?

> *Ellen, 37, knows how great it is. "I've been jogging for a few years but I was getting more and more worn out from it, partly because I was having a lot of discomfort in my hips. Now I enter mini-marathons, and keeping up with my husband is no trouble at all."*

CORE BENEFITS

You *can* enjoy all the benefits described above, and more, if you will give fifteen minutes a day to performing the Core exercise program I've used with such success for the women I treat in my practice. Moving through your busy life with a strong and supple and pain-free body is your right—because that is how nature intended you to be. I'm going to show you how to restore to your body what your life as a woman saps from it.

WHY I WROTE THIS BOOK

One morning a few years ago, I was on my way to work. As I stood, surrounded by other riders on a slow-moving bus, I started to observe how some of the women aboard carried themselves. I've had this habit for a long time. Even before I became a physical therapist I was always fascinated by the way people—and especially women—held, and moved, their bodies.

A well-dressed, fit woman in her forties who was standing next to me kept tugging at the strap of her obviously overloaded carryall. Her whole body leaned so far to the right it seemed as though the carryall had a gravitational pull all its own. Near her, a woman in her twenties, who was sitting, tilted her head to an extreme angle as she talked on a cell phone. She continually rubbed her neck, which was obviously hurting. Then there was the tall thirtyish woman who carried fatigue around her shoulders like a heavy shawl. Her whole body slumped forward as she held on to the back of a seat with both hands.

What a shame, I thought to myself. *These women look so uncomfortable—and they don't have to be.*

Then, as the bus stalled in traffic, I noticed a woman on the street, who was at least eighty years old. In sharp contrast to the women on the bus, all of them much younger than she, this woman carried herself with freedom and ease. As she strode confidently on her way, her body was in perfect alignment. Looking at her, I realized how much I could do for the women on the bus—and every woman.

My work could give them the gift of strength and easy movement and physical balance today, and for the rest of their lives. They too would look, and move, like that confident, graceful, strong woman on the street, no matter what their age.

I decided right then that I would write a book that would enable women to use everything I had learned through my work, and that this book would be my way of fulfilling the commitment I had made, after my mother's early death from a heart attack, to the cause of women's health. I want to help women to change their lives, starting at the core. And I know how to do it quickly, easily, and inexpensively.

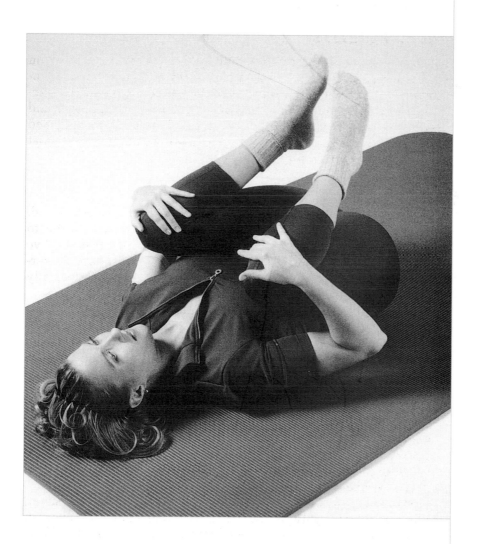

fifteen minutes a day
that will change your life

The Core Program is the fifteen-minutes-a-day, five-times-a-week exercise regimen that will give you benefits no single other fitness program can offer. In a very short time it will:

- Build strength
- Abolish muscle aches and pains
- Improve your posture
- Put an end to joint stiffness
- Give you a graceful, easy stride
- Eliminate fatigue after each session
- Relax your body so that you get a good night's sleep
- Improve your balance
- Enhance your stamina for the day ahead
- Heighten your sexual pleasure
- Rid you of occasional nausea and headaches and other symptoms for which doctors can find no cause

In fact, from your very first workout, you will experience an increased sense of well-being—a new sense of ease, energy and relief from everyday aches and pains.

The Core Program will give your body a head-to-toe workout that will also tone your muscles and carve inches off your waist and hips. You'll look great and feel terrific. Best of all, the easy-to-do Core movements can be done no matter how old you are. It doesn't matter whether you are overweight or skinny, fit or sedentary. Maybe you'll be able to do only one or two to start, but eventually almost everyone is able to perform all the exercises in the Core Foundation. Many others will go on to the more advanced versions of the program.

All you need is an exercise mat, which stores easily under a bed, or simply use a large folded towel for cushioning. Wear an outfit that allows you easy movement. Sweats are fine; so is an old leotard or leggings and a T-shirt. After you master the Core Foundation program, you have the option of continuing to the Intermediate program, and eventually to the Ultimate Core. These more advanced programs include some new exercises, and some variations on the Foundation exercises. They also introduce the use of simple hand and ankle weights, for added benefits.

I know that being a woman equals being busy. Family. Career. Children. Friends. Shopping. Traveling. Cooking. Grooming. Gardening. Cleaning. Exercise. And this is only a partial list. With two children (one a baby), two physical therapy offices and one husband, my life is extremely hectic. So hectic, in fact, that I barely managed to do the photo shoot for the exercise sections of this book before I got really big with the pregnancy for my second child. I was three months pregnant when we did these photo sessions, as may be obvious in some of the pictures. So I think I understand as well as anyone how precious, and how short, time is. That's why I made sure that the Core Program is lifestyle-friendly.

Do the program when it is convenient for you, in the privacy of your home or as part of your gym workout. Do it in the morning, the evening, or anytime in between. (I have patients who close their office doors and take a restorative fifteen-minute Core "break" in the afternoon.)

AS A WOMAN, YOU NEED THE CORE PROGRAM

The Core Program derives from my experience of treating thousands of women for the most frequent aches and pains they experienced in their heads, necks, shoulders, arms, backs and legs. I noticed that, no matter where they were feeling discomfort, all of their problems seemed to relate to underdeveloped and unbalanced muscle groups in one area of the body—the core. What I'm calling the "core" is the torso, which extends from the base of the neck to the bottom of the spine, and includes the abdomen and all the back and hip muscles. These are the parts that stabilize as well as encase the vertebrae surrounding the spinal cord, through which the thirty-one pairs of spinal nerves branching off from the spinal cord emerge.

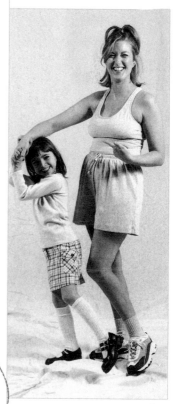

The brachial plexus is the group of nerves that branches off the spinal cord through the area of the neck, extending into the upper extremities of the body. The sciatic nerve, the largest nerve in your body, which is actually made up of a group of five nerve roots, emerges from the lumbar spine and passes through the buttocks and down each leg, supplying the lower extremities of the body. Because their ultimate source is the spinal cord, the nerves in both your arms and your legs function best when you have a strong and stable core.

Both the neck and the lower back are dependent on the core muscles to stabilize the spine so that all the vertebral segments align with one another in a way that does not compress the nerves that pass through them. When nerves are compressed they can't deliver full electrical impulses to muscles. When that happens, the muscles can't work the way they should. Weakness and pain are the result.

SOAS muscle Runs over Hips + FRont of upper THIGHS

Very Important

7

In almost all of the patients I was seeing, I found that the core muscles supporting the torso weren't as strong as they needed to be—and that was the root of the discomfort.

The exercises I give to my patients—the exercises of the Core Program, which are the same exercises I'll be giving to you in this book—strengthen the core muscles. When those muscles are strong, discomfort disappears, and as long as you keep doing the program, it won't come back. Working the core muscles also helps to keep your body in good alignment, so that sitting and walking and running are easier.

There is a clear cause and effect. The stronger the core, the better the body works. Just as a firm infrastructure supports a building and prevents it from breaking down inside, a reinforced core becomes the basis of a strong, supported body.

That's why it made great sense to me to write a book offering a series of exercises specially designed to strengthen the core—and to gear it to women. As women facing women's challenges, we need to do what is necessary to make sure our bodies function smoothly throughout our lives. As I'll discuss in more detail in chapter two, there are numerous lifestyle stresses and strains that are unique to women, as well as physical demands on us, none of which we can do much to change. What we *can* change is how we respond to them. It's imperative that we take charge of how we use our bodies, which is what the Core Program can help us to do—and the earlier we make these changes, the better.

I always ask my patients if they would risk waiting until they were age 65 to fund a retirement account. After they look at me dumbfounded for a moment, they all reply with an indignant "No!" The same conclusion applies to meeting the needs of your body. Doing the Core Program is like investing in a retirement plan for your health. Start it now, and watch those dividends roll in. You'll be able to live your life to the fullest. You'll also find that the more you do the Core Program, the more effortless it becomes. I've been doing it for so long, it's as automatic as brushing my teeth.

Ultimately, the Core Program does something no other fitness plan can do: It makes you resilient against the "normal deterioration" of age.

THE MISSING FITNESS LINK: A CORE PROGRAM TO COMPLEMENT OTHER FITNESS REGIMENS

If you are doing either aerobics or weight training or both, you might think that the exercise you are already doing, along with nutritious food and supplements, is all you need to keep your body in good condition. But that's not true. Please don't misunderstand me: I strongly support both aerobic exercise and weight training, as well as eating a balanced diet and drinking plenty of water, of course.

However, these healthy choices can't give your body the strength, balance and alignment it requires to perform hundreds of daily actions effortlessly, and without any kind of physical discomfort. Nor can other fitness programs prevent injuries—much less relieve pain.

Only the core exercises can enable your skeleton, muscles and joints to work together optimally, because only the core exercises offer the unique combination of strengthening, stretching, balancing and realigning that allows your body to withstand daily wear and tear.

However, you may choose, as many of my patients do, to add the Core Program to other workouts. Whether you quietly practice yoga, take part in boisterous aerobics classes and/or do strenuous weight training, the core exercises will give you a complementary program that will make your other fitness efforts more effective. These terrific movements will align and strengthen your body to prevent the injuries that often occur in other exercise programs. Even if you are just planning to begin a walking routine, doing the Core Program first will help you build your muscles properly, thereby preventing the muscle strains and pains you might otherwise suffer, especially if you haven't done any exercise in a long time.

Bodywork Techniques: Help, Not a Cure

Many patients who come to me have tried many of the bodywork techniques that are so popular today. All offer some benefits—and a few present some significant drawbacks. Here are some you may recognize:

The Alexander Technique and **Feldenkrais,** which both feature gentle and rhythmical balance-related movements. Unfortunately, they both lack strength-building components.

Pilates, which is excellent at strength-building, muscle-balancing and alignment. But to use Pilates equipment you have to go to a Pilates studio, usually paying for individual instruction. You can also go to mat classes, but it's hard to master the Pilates techniques without one-on-one attention.

Massage therapy, which helps to relax people while easing muscle soreness, but does nothing for strength. Also, it's not something you can do yourself. In order to get the temporary restorative benefits of massage therapy, you have to pay for the services of a massage therapist.

Tai chi, which focuses on weight shifting and is good for stability, balance and strength. However, the movements of tai chi neither strengthen the arms nor open the spaces between vertebrae so that nerves can avoid becoming impinged.

Yoga, which increases muscle flexibility but doesn't build core muscle strength. It can also overstretch and thereby weaken certain muscles, resulting in imbalances in opposing muscle groups.

Only the movements of the Core Program deliver relaxation *and* muscle building *and* flexibility *and* body realignment. No formal instruction or instructor is necessary, and there is no risk of injury.

A PHYSICAL THERAPIST'S APPROACH TO PHYSICAL FITNESS

I understand how a woman's body can safely achieve fitness because, unlike most other fitness experts, I received in-depth hands-on medical training. I took four years of premed courses in college, where I majored in biology. Then for two years I attended a physical therapy school that was part of the University of Medicine and Dentistry of New Jersey, before attaining my degree. I have also done extensive study of the musculoskeletal system in advanced postgraduate courses.

When a patient comes to see me, I use my training as a physical therapist to evaluate her in a particular way. Besides listening to her description of pain and dysfunction, I determine the range of motion of various joints and perform a thorough manual muscle test to assess the strength of all the major muscle groups.

As a physical therapist, I assess a woman's body from head to toe. I know every muscle and joint and can pinpoint areas that need help. I know how to exercise muscles in order to balance them. And I know how to put the joints in alignment, which allows the bones to bear weight as they should, while eliminating any strain on your joints. But I don't just heal injuries. I work with my patients to show them how to prevent future injuries—that's part of my job. I can help women regain strength—without joint injury—in seconds. (See the box on page 12.)

After treating thousands of patients, I can confidently say that there is a recognizable pattern of muscle weakness and tightness that leads to almost all of the common injuries I see. Knowing what has worked well for my patients has enabled me to design a series of exercises to strengthen what tends to get weak and stretch what tends to get tight. This is why the Core Program's effects go beyond mere fitness—they will affect your ability to feel well and function at maximum capacity throughout your life.

While fitness experts can make your muscles strong, they don't look at a woman's body the way I do. Their advice to lift weights to build bone mass makes excellent sense, but they often lack the expertise they need to teach you how to do it in a way that won't harm your joints. And they are unable to address the underlying causes of achiness and fatigue.

I've been a physical therapist for nearly fifteen years. I love what I do for a very simple reason: Every day I work with patients who get better. The smile I often see on a woman's face after just a couple of minutes of treatment tells me she is on her way to feeling great. And that gives me tremendous gratification. I see tension melt away along with aches and pains. I see changes in bodies as women learn to move themselves in more efficient ways. Best of all, I get to listen every day to women who tell me that they feel better than ever before, and that they have found a new trust in their bodies and new hope for the future.

Making such life-improving changes is a huge accomplishment for anyone, but more than a few of the women I treat are recovering from severe injuries and complicated surgical procedures. A number of them are referred to me by physicians at several major New York City medical centers, including the Hospital for Special Surgery, St. Luke's–Roosevelt Hospital Center, NYU Medical Center, New York–Presbyterian, and the University Hospitals of Columbia and Cornell.

My work introduces me to all kinds of interesting people of all ages. In my private practice, I treat children under 10 as well as grandparents over 90. In my waiting room people who haven't exercised in years share sofa space with Olympic athletes. Business people, including top executives from Fortune 500 companies, regularly arrive at my Manhattan office. I also operate a second Brill Physical Therapy office on-site at Morgan Stanley for employees of the company and their families.

On occasion, I travel to my patients. I've been to Beijing to help a high-level government official who had suffered from chronic back pain, and several times a year I fly to North Carolina to take care of the coach and players of the nationally ranked men's basketball team at Duke University.

Still, much of my work is focused on the musculoskeletal systems of women who are probably just like you. They have vague aches and pains that doctors can't explain, or they have minor injuries that have occurred while doing exercise or playing a sport. Included among the common injuries I see are herniated discs; rotator cuff tears; tennis elbow; all kinds of neck and back pain; bursitis/tendinitis (which is inflammation from overuse) in the hip, shoulder and knee; cartilage and ACL (anterior cruciate ligament) knee tears; chondromalacia (dull aching pain behind the kneecap); sprains and strains; Morton's neuroma; hammertoes; bunions; heels spurs; and plantar fascitis (inflammation of the plantar fascia, the connective tissue on the bottom of the feet). By the way, age does not necessarily contribute to these injuries. Thirteen-year-olds get them just as adults do.

But no matter what injuries I am treating, my work centers on

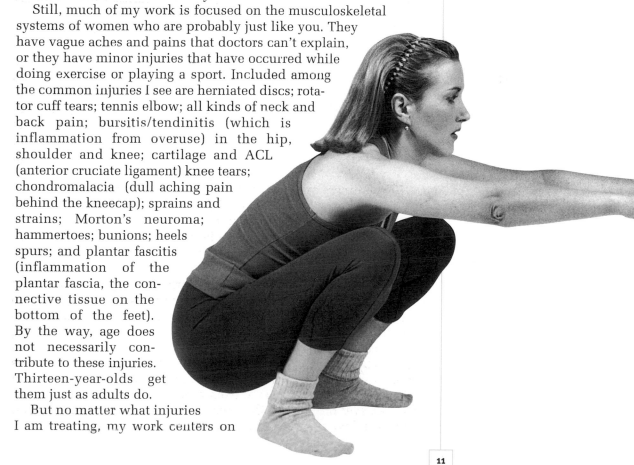

building up and protecting the core of the body, because all these injuries are caused or made worse by core muscles that aren't as strong as they need to be.

THE FIRST CORE GOALS: STRENGTH AND TONING, BALANCE AND ALIGNMENT

My female-centered regimen goes to the heart of what women need to function well and feel as good as they possibly can. I'll show you how to work *with* your body, not against it. Instead of feeling weighed down by fatigued muscles, you'll get a burst of energy that will give you a lift. Knowing you can depend on your body, and watching it become better toned and defined within a few months, will give you a whole new level of confidence.

To make all these wonderful things happen, the Core Program will:

REBALANCE YOUR MUSCLES

Unlike other fitness routines, the Core Program restores balance between muscles that work as a couple. The job of muscles is to pull, either concentrically (by creating force through shortening), or eccentrically (by absorbing force through elongating). But, as is the case with many couples, often one muscle becomes more dominant than the other. When this happens, their relationship is not equal. The result is that the muscles don't work in harmony, and the joint they attach to suffers.

Think of it this way: The muscle couples work like a seesaw, with the joint they attach to being the axis of motion. When that seesaw goes up and down in a constant, equal motion, the joint is where it should be. It's the same way in your body. There must be balance between muscles in order for them, and the joints attached to them, to work efficiently and painlessly. If there's an imbalance, problems can occur.

For instance, if you slouch, over a period of time the pectoral muscles in your chest will shorten, and become dominant. Over time, the upper back muscles with which they are paired will become elongated, or stretched. Then it becomes more difficult for the back muscles to pull with equal force. And here's an example of what can then go wrong: You want to push a heavy door open, but when you move your shoulder, your dominant pectoral muscles kick in before the upper back muscles with which they are paired. This imbalance alters the force on the shoulder joint, and can lead to injury. If you strain to push open a door and you feel pain in your shoulder, it means that your pectoral and back muscles are not balanced and your shoulder joint is out of alignment.

RELEASE MUSCLE TENSION

Muscles that have shortened feel tense. By stretching short muscles, you can release tension and experience an immediate feeling of relaxation.

Instant Strength Booster

This simple yet incredibly effective neck retraction will boost your strength in seconds as it relieves tension in neck muscles. The movement expands the spaces between vertebrae so nerves in the upper extremities are free to send electrical impulses to muscles in the hands and arms. The muscles, in turn, can generate more force. (This is the same thing you do in the first movement of the first exercise in the Core Foundation, the Head-to-Toe Prep.) You can do this anytime, anywhere.

THE MOVEMENT

- Sit, or stand, straight.
- Slide your head back, tuck your chin so that the back of your neck is elongated and your ears are over your shoulders, and pull your shoulder blades together. Hold the position for three seconds.
- Release slowly to a relaxed position.
- Repeat six times.

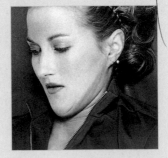

STRENGTHEN MUSCLES WITHOUT BULKING UP THE BODY

Moving the body against gravity reinforces muscles. The more you do the exercises, the more they will define your muscles, thereby toning your body and giving it a sleek look.

ENHANCE STAMINA

Deep breathing, an integral part of the Core Program, delivers oxygen to muscles, which gives them endurance while also helping to relieve muscle tension.

RESHAPE YOUR BODY

You'll tone your abdomen, hips and buttocks and give your arms better definition, too. Inches will disappear even without dieting because the more muscle you have, the more fat your body will burn. You'll be enhancing your lean muscle mass. If you are on a weight loss plan, doing the exercises will give you an extra boost.

RESTORE ALIGNMENT

By stretching muscles that are shortened, and strengthening muscles that are weak, your joints will be restored to their optimal position. This means that your skeletal alignment will be reestablished. With your joints in their optimal positions, you will sit, stand and walk tall and strong and move with ease. Your posture will improve, allowing you to move more gracefully.

INCREASE FLEXIBILITY

The flexibility of both muscles and joints is augmented. Achieving optimal muscle flexibility allows joints to move through their normal range of motion.

INCREASE CAPACITY FOR SEXUAL PLEASURE

Because the core exercises strengthen the pelvic floor muscles, which include the muscles that contract during orgasm, you may discover a surprising side benefit—easier-to-reach, more intense orgasms.

THE SECOND CORE GOAL: PREVENTION

You may believe that aging will take an inevitable toll on your body. Perhaps you've already begun to notice that when you go to the gym you are having a problem with urinary stress incontinence—"leaking," in more colloquial terms. This condition afflicts many women, especially as they get older.

Or if either arthritis or osteoporosis runs in your family, you might be concerned that you will eventually have to cope with one of these conditions. Perhaps you look at your grandmother and wonder whether you too will morph into a weaker version of your former self.

I'm happy to tell you that these scenarios do not have to happen. While a woman's body goes through inevitable physical changes over the years, age by itself doesn't determine how well a woman moves or holds herself nor does it dictate how strong or how healthy she is. There's a lot you can do to help prevent arthritis and osteoporosis as well as many other problems.

The Core Program will:

REDUCE THE RISK OF DEVELOPING OSTEOARTHRITIS, OR RELIEVE THE SYMPTOMS

This painful joint inflammation, which stems from either overuse or underuse, can be avoided. When joints are in their normal alignment they absorb the forces exerted against them without injury. When joints are balanced they are lubricated, because the synovial fluid that is secreted by the membrane surrounding the joints isn't cut off by any kind of compression. A balanced joint is friction-free and healthy, allowing for ease of movement.

> *Sarah, who had chronic knee pain from arthritis, made great progress once she started doing the core exercises. "Walking down steps was so painful and I was getting worse. I just couldn't accept that, at 32, I was going to lose mobility. With the Core Program the pain disappeared, my strength returned and now I'm in really good physical shape."*

REDUCE THE RISK OF DEVELOPING OSTEOPOROSIS, OR RELIEVE THE SYMPTOMS

The core exercises cause muscles to pull on bone, which prompts the production of new bone cells. You can actually help create more bone mass by doing these movements. This is very important, as a decrease of just 10 percent in bone mass can result in 50 to 100 percent greater incidence of fracture. Bone density tests, which measure standard deviations from peak bone mass, have shown genuine changes in patients whom I have put on this exercise regimen.

> *Ana, who at 80 had osteoporosis, was amazed at the differences in her body. "I gained one whole point in bone density since I was tested last year. In addition, I can move so much better than I did before. After three months on the Core Program I could turn my head from side to side without a problem—and that's something I hadn't been able to do in much too long."*

DECREASE OR ELIMINATE THE INCIDENCE OF URINARY STRESS INCONTINENCE

The same muscles that contract during orgasm can stop the flow of urine. So in building up the muscles of the pelvic floor, which hold the pubic bone and tailbone in place, you will also be helping to prevent urinary stress incontinence. The muscles of the bladder are strengthened as well.

AVERT INJURIES

Muscle weakness leads to injury. When a demand is put on your body that you can't meet—whether it is lifting weights or lifting a child, taking an aerobics class or running to catch a bus, even sitting at a computer all day—injuries happen. But when your musculoskeletal system is strong and well balanced, you are much less likely to hurt yourself.

THE THIRD CORE GOAL: MAKING SENSE OF DISCOMFORT

I've heard so many variations on this theme. Perhaps you are bothered by an ache in your side that just won't go away. After a couple of weeks the bloating and distress prompt you to make an appointment with your doctor. After looking you over, she recommends a few diagnostic tests. When they come back normal and you tell her you're still not feeling right, she recommends one or more invasive tests. (It is critical not to overlook a potentially serious condition. All my patients have proper screening to rule out any pathology causing uncommon pain.)

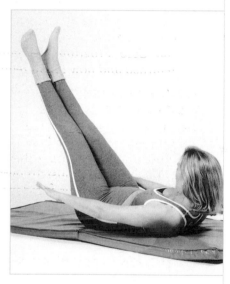

One week and a couple thousand dollars later, you get the great news: There's nothing wrong with you. But, while you heave a sigh of relief, you still don't feel very good. The physician's suggestion to try to minimize stress seems like a good idea, but you wonder if that will really help what is bothering you.

From your doctor's point of view, "something wrong" means a clearly defined illness or injury. These are the organic dysfunctions mainstream medicine looks for and knows how to treat. Unfortunately, when no such problem can be detected by tests, the patient falls into a "gray" area. What is bothering you is caused by a problem outside the doctor's range of expertise.

If this is the situation you find yourself in, my program may be able to give you the help you need. Many "gray" problems are caused by a problem at the core—which is my area of expertise.

First, take the self-tests on pages 27–31 to determine whether your core muscles are weak. Then start doing the Core Foundation exercises and stick with them for at least three weeks. In as little time as a week you'll start to feel better and experience major reductions in discomfort—and a major boost in energy and well-being. And soon you will discover that you want to keep doing the exercises, so that you can keep enjoying their benefits for as long as you live.

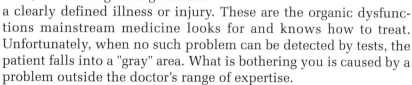

This is a program that women of all ages can use. Even if you're so weak that all you can do at first is the Head-to-Toe Prep, you'll find it worthwhile.

THE FOURTH CORE GOAL: PROVIDING RELIEF FROM INJURY AND ILLNESS

In addition to treating all kinds of sports injuries, I have had great success in helping patients with many types of physical disorders. If you have any of the following chronic or even life-threatening ailments, the core exercises can boost your available strength and stamina.

Carpal tunnel syndrome
Cancer, including postmastectomy
Diastasis recti
Fibromyalgia
Hiatal hernia
Lymphedema
Lupus
Rheumatoid arthritis
Scleroderma

Monica, 52, who was diagnosed with fibromyalgia three years ago, has benefited greatly from the Core Program. "I began with the first exercise of the Core Program—the Head-to-Toe Prep—and did it for three weeks. Then I was able to do the rest of the exercises—I could even do them twice a day! Before I started the exercises I could sit and work for only two hours; the pain in my shoulders and hips was that bad. Now I have a lot more stamina—and comfort."

THE CORE RESULTS

In addition to getting quick relief from aches and pains, my patients have reported better digestion, reduced bloating, more refreshing sleep—and even better sex! Add an improved ability to relax and you have everything you need to feel great.

I am also going to give you, a woman just like myself, a formula for well-being that includes:

- a head-to-toe workout you will not find in any other book
- information you need about avoiding the potentially harmful recommendations found in many other books and exercise videos
- a program to help keep building strength and flexibility, even as you grow older
- the facts about what injuries women are most likely to suffer and what you can do to prevent them
- the means to relieving physical stress, pain and discomfort that has no underlying pathological cause

- confirmation that those aches and pains are not "all in your head"—even if traditional medicine doesn't acknowledge them
- the reassurance that you can feel better than ever with each passing year

Ultimately, when someone asks you how you feel, you won't hesitate to answer, "I feel great, right down to the core!"

BEFORE YOU BEGIN

If you're eager to start the Core Program, you can go directly to chapter seven, "The Core Foundation," which is the basic program I give to all my patients. Even if you pass all the self-tests, do the Foundation program for a minimum of one week before progressing to the Intermediate Core.

If you didn't pass all the self-tests, I recommend doing the Core Foundation for three weeks. After that, you can, if you wish to increase the intensity of the workout, progress to the Intermediate Core, which is described in chapter eight. Then, after another three weeks, if you feel you can do all those exercises with ease, you can opt for the Ultimate Core, the most intense version of the Core Program, described in chapter nine.

If you'd like more information about the science behind the Core Program, how I arrived at it and how to get psyched for doing it, read the following chapters, too:

In chapter three, I'll tell you about my own physical journey, which led me to the Core Program.

In chapter four, I'll talk about posture and how the Core Program helps to realign the body.

In chapter five, I'll give you an easy-to-follow owner's manual to your musculoskeletal system.

Then, right before the Core Programs begin, I'll provide a section on how to motivate yourself to get started. After you've begun, you won't need any motivational pep talks. The way you feel will provide you all the motivation you need!

Following the Core Program chapters, you'll find two more:

Chapter ten shows you the best way to perform the weight-training exercises that many women do in addition to the Core. These exercises can enhance the effectiveness of the Core Program—and vice versa—if you do them correctly. But they can also cause injuries if you don't. And then there are exercises that shouldn't be done at all—especially by women. This chapter gives you lots of gym "do's" and "don'ts" to make your workouts safe and maximally beneficial.

Finally, there's a question-and-answer chapter based on queries I've gotten from many of my patients, which will probably clarify issues you've been wondering about, too.

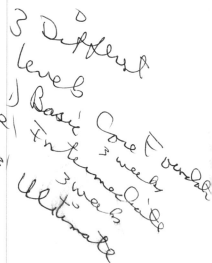

3 Different levels
1) Basic Core Foundation
2) Intermediate 3 weeks
3) Ultimate 3 weeks

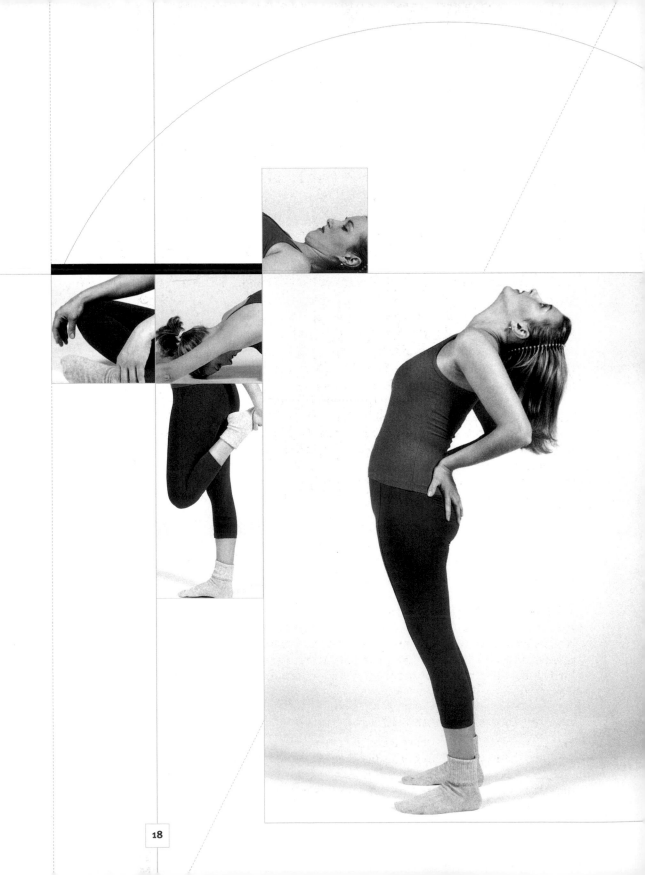

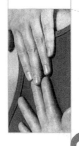

different to the core

A WOMAN TO THE CORE

The women I see in my practice range in age from their early twenties to late eighties. They're of all shapes and sizes, and all degrees of fitness, too.

A number of them work out frequently; others intend to start exercising "someday." Some are ultra-thin, others carry extra weight, and most fall somewhere in between. Yet they all share something in common that irrevocably separates them from men.

Women have a unique *physical core,* thanks to the reproductive system and its hormones, which affects the alignment of their bones and joints, and also dictates a pattern of muscle distribution that is very different from men's.

Women also have a distinctive *lifestyle core,* which results in a variety of behaviors that directly affect the musculoskeletal system—often in ways that present special challenges to endurance, stamina and the ability to withstand injury.

The Female Physical Core

It is no secret that men and women have very different bodies. Nonetheless, you may be unaware of the impact of some of these differences. The fact that nature shaped a woman's body for childbirth has some surprising effects on her musculoskeletal system. These effects first become evident as a girl reaches puberty.

THE PELVIC DIFFERENCE

Maybe it doesn't sound very scientific to say that your hip bone is connected to your thighbone, and your thighbone is connected to your knee bone, etc., but the fact is, your knee is a hinge joint, and the way it absorbs force changes whenever the alignment of the bones above and below it changes.

As soon as you had your first menstrual period, you began to develop pelvic curves that directly affected the alignment of your knees. First of all, your pelvis widened. When that happened, your gluteal muscles became stretched and lost some of their power. At the same time their opposing muscles became tighter, which rotated your thigh bone inward.

When that happened, your kneecaps shifted outward, so that any bending of the knee, such as when you walked down steps, caused the kneecaps to move out of their normal alignment over the second toes. Once the knee motion shifted, your ankles lost mobility, which forced the midfoot to compensate. This, in turn, flattened your arches.

As an adolescent you took part in gym exercises in school, which was good. Unfortunately, some of the exercises didn't take your physical changes into account and unwittingly perpetuated faulty movement patterns. If you played basketball, for example, the running and jumping exerted forces equal to three times your body weight on your lower extremities. (When you walk your knees absorb forces up to one and a half times your body weight.) Not surprisingly, any existing muscular imbalances you had were stressed—unless these imbalances were addressed with proper exercises.

If you began to experience injuries that limited your participation in sports, now you know why: Weak hip and gluteal muscles could have been causing your recurring knee problems.

The Core Program takes the effect of your pelvic differences as a woman into consideration. In doing so it helps to prevent lower extremity injuries and to counteract years of accumulated knee stress. The exercises stabilize joints by working muscles that surround and support each joint.

THE HORMONAL DIFFERENCES

A woman's hormones provide the script for the exquisitely fine-tuned biological program that enables her to bear children. Obviously, her body is expressly designed to get pregnant and give birth and breastfeed. But the same hormones that make these functions possible have surprising effects on other body systems, too.

Hormones play an important role where muscle is concerned, for example. Women have comparatively high levels of estrogen and low levels of testosterone, while men have comparatively low levels of estrogen and high levels of testosterone. Since testosterone stimulates muscle growth, men have more muscle mass than women do. Yet women need muscle strength, which is one of the reasons why women in particular can benefit from the muscle-strengthening offered by the Core Program.

Hormones affect joint laxity, too. As explained in the discussion of knee injuries, women have looser ligaments than men, which are even looser during ovulation. The fact that women have looser lig-

The Ovulation-Knee Connection

Research is beginning to look at the possible connection between ovulation and the incidence of knee injury. With the number of young female athletes increasing all the time, definitive studies need to be done. However, a study published in the *Journal of Orthopedic Research* reported a fascinating finding. Researchers in California observed forty women with ACL (anterior cruciate ligament) knee tears. They found that a high number of their subjects suffered their injuries during the ovulation phase of their menstrual cycles. This phase is marked by a significant rise in estrogen, as well as another hormone called relaxin. Ligaments, the ropelike structures that stabilize joints by attaching bones to bones, tend to be looser in women than in men. During ovulation, the hormones cause ligaments to relax even more. Because the ligaments may become too loose to maintain the stability of the joint, they become more vulnerable to tearing. And, unlike muscles, ligaments can't be changed through exercise.

aments means that women's joints are more flexible than those of men; it also means they have to rely more on muscle strength to keep their joints in good alignment. Having stronger muscles will make for more stable joints, which means both fewer injuries and greater ease of motion.

Other hormone-related differences between men and women relate directly to their reproductive systems. The core exercises will enhance the health and well-being of a woman's reproductive system in several ways: They will help strengthen muscles that have to bear the additional weight of pregnancy, and will relieve back and foot pain stemming from already weak and imbalanced muscles that are further strained by pregnancy. The exercises will also strengthen the pelvic muscles so important in childbirth, thereby making labor and delivery easier.

The hormonal changes that occur in women over the course of the life cycle also point to the need for my Core Program. For example, while estrogen may not do much for muscles, it's terrific for bones (and not to mention hearts!). Using exercise to maximize the benefits of estrogen during the menstruating years will mean that you have maximum amounts of bone mass to draw upon when menopause begins, bringing with it a decrease in estrogen levels, which in turn leads to an acceleration of bone loss and a higher risk of osteoporosis.

Another common effect of the estrogen depletion that occurs at menopause is that the muscles of the pelvic floor, which are responsible for supporting the function of the bladder, vagina and rectum, lose what is called their "fluffiness," which is another way of saying their tone or elasticity. If the muscles of the pelvic floor don't maintain their tone, urinary incontinence problems, as well as decreased sexual satisfaction, can be the result, as discussed earlier.

The Core Program will help reinforce the benefits of estrogen and counteract many of the deficits that may occur when estrogen levels fall at menopause. The core exercises will help optimize the bone-building that continues to occur from birth until women reach their mid-twenties, so that they'll have a plentiful supply of bone to draw upon in later years; will help maintain that bone density until age 35, which is when most women begin losing more bone than they are able to build; and will put the brakes on the acceleration of bone loss that occurs at menopause and during the years afterward.

The Core Program also strengthens the muscles of the pelvic floor, which will help women at all stages of life.

THE MUSCLE DISTRIBUTION DIFFERENCE

Nature determined that females house comparatively more muscle in the lower half of their bodies, and less in the upper half. While pound for pound women have as much leg power, they do not have as much upper-body strength. But they experience as many if not more demands on that strength as men do, thanks to the unique demands of their daily lives, as we'll be discussing below—not to mention the fact that they have breasts, which add extra weight for the upper body to carry.

My Core Program targets the muscles of the upper torso, which are in particular need of strengthening in women. Doing these exercises will help you be stronger and better able to meet the demands of daily life, while also protecting you from injury.

The Female Lifestyle Core

As women we react differently than men to the world in which we live, and these behaviors have a direct impact on our bodies. These distinctions can be seen in how we:

- cope with stress
- lose and gain weight
- carry bags, kids and other assorted "stuff"

A DIFFERENT RESPONSE TO STRESS: A TENDENCY TO TENSE

When confronted by stressful situations, all human beings, men and women alike, undergo a sequence of physiological events, which are part of their built-in stress reaction system, popularly known as the "fight or flight" response.

You know what that feels like. Something happens to alarm or upset you, and your heart races, your palms sweat. Muscles tense while adrenaline, released from the adrenal gland, pours into your bloodstream. Blood pumps to muscles as well as organs—like the heart and the eyes—whose heightened activity is needed for immediate survival. Nature is preparing you to either confront an enemy or escape it. Your sympathetic nervous system, which causes all these reactions, is on high alert.

While both men—and women—undergo the same "fight or flight" response, they react to stress in different ways. Ever see two men get into a fender bender? Did they speak calmly and civilly as they assessed the damage to their cars and exchanged insurance information? Put two men in a stress-filled situation and stand back. At the very least a heated verbal exchange is pretty much assured. Once that anger is externalized their sympathetic nervous systems usually turn "off." Something different happens with women.

Women tend not to express their anger openly; instead, they internalize it, with the result that they feel its effects long after the "fight or flight" moment has passed. So in the minutes and hours afterward, muscles that were already tense tighten even more.

The Core Program will deliver benefits from early in a woman's life straight through to menopause and on to old age. It can help young women build their supplies not only of bone but of muscle, so that they will be better equipped to feel and look good now, and to defend themselves against the encroachment of age in the years to come. Do you know that women lose muscle mass at the rate of 1 percent for each year over the age of 40 unless they are doing weight-training, which involves the use of free weights and/or the kind of weight-training machines usually found at a gym—*or they are performing exercises that use body weight as resistance against gravity, as the Core Program exercises do.*

When muscles tense, they clamp down on nerves within them. The nerves, whose job it is to deliver the electrical impulses that allow the muscle to work properly, are entrapped. Consequently, electrical impulses from the nerves don't get through to the muscle and muscle weakness, spasms or pain may be the direct result.

Furthermore, because blood vessels are compressed when muscles tense, the muscles don't receive an adequate blood supply, which deprives them of oxygen and nutrients, which every cell needs to function.

When this happens over and over again, the natural contraction and relaxation of the muscle is disrupted. It's easy to identify a muscle experiencing an electrical "short circuit" and a disrupted blood supply: It hurts, it's weak and it doesn't work the way it should.

In women, tension is typically felt in the neck, back, shoulders and the jaw and face. Headaches and fatigue are common symptoms. And some women eventually develop TMJ (temporomandibular joint) disorder, with symptoms that may include painful grinding of the teeth, facial pain, headaches and ringing in the ears. (Interestingly enough, men tend to feel tension in the chest, pelvis, hips and buttocks.)

My Core Program relaxes tense muscles, which results in better nerve transmission and blood circulation. The way you experience the result is that you simply feel more relaxed. A deep-breathing component of the program enhances oxygen uptake—which also makes you feel more relaxed.

WEIGHT FLUCTUATIONS

If there is a woman who hasn't watched her weight vary by at least ten pounds during her adult years, I haven't met her. There are so many reasons why a woman's weight can fluctuate. Some women put on a few premenstrual pounds each month and quickly lose them. Others gain dozens of pounds during pregnancies and never manage to lose them after giving birth.

A traumatic event can trigger a substantial weight gain—or loss. A happy occasion can add some pounds since, as a society, we use food as a form of celebration. But an ecstatic experience, like falling in love for the first time, can cause weight to drop, because the woman may be too excited to eat much.

Dieting also plays a big role in our lives. Pick up virtually any women's magazine and you'll see the newest regimen promising a quick way to achieve an "ideal" shape. Yo-yo dieting is a particularly female form of behavior. While men do, of course, gain and lose weight (and take off pounds faster than women because their increased muscle mass burns more calories), they don't usually put on and lose pounds in a yo-yo cycle.

This up-and-down sequence puts a lot of physical stress on the body.

Carrying extra poundage will make an existing imbalance worse. Remember your pelvic curves? When you gain weight any muscular imbalance you already have will worsen. Your feet will roll in even more, putting more stress on your knee joints. Being ten pounds overweight can increase the likelihood of developing arthritis in the knees by 50 percent. Maintaining a strong and straight body can become harder to do.

When a woman is too thin, however, she increases her risk for developing osteoporosis. Her highly restricted caloric intake doesn't supply enough calcium. Also, her smaller mass of muscles and soft tissues can contribute to reduced bone mass. And because fat cells produce smaller than normal amounts of the hormone estrogen, emaciated women may stop ovulating, further increasing the risk of osteoporosis.

Without consistently healthy eating habits that help assure normal weight and give your body the fuel it needs, your muscles and bones will suffer.

The Core Program boosts your musculoskeletal system whatever your weight. If you are carrying some extra pounds, these exercises will not stress your joints. If you are ultra-thin, they can help increase your bone mass.

LUGGING TOO MUCH "STUFF"

A man puts a wallet in his pocket. Sometimes he carries a briefcase or throws on a backpack. A woman will load herself down with several varieties of "excess baggage" at one time. My grandmother left Scotland with less "baggage" than I carry on a daily basis. A heavy handbag, a portfolio, groceries, shopping bags, a diaper bag, a stroller, not to mention the child who goes in the stroller! The list goes on and on. In the course of a day the average woman lifts and hauls a substantial amount of weight.

Carrying heavy loads adds strain to already imbalanced muscles. And think about which part of the body bears all that weight. Generally speaking, it's the upper body that is most in need of strengthening. Moreover, it's likely that you favor one side of your body over the other. If you always carry your shoulder bag on one side of your body, as most women do, the muscles on the other side of your body will be less developed and you'll suffer the results of a muscle imbalance. The muscles that do all the work will shorten from all the contracting they do, while the muscles on the other side will become long and weak.

The Core Program balances your muscles and restores them to their optimal length, which enables them to do their work effectively—and without stress, strain, injury or pain. You'll be able to do what you need to do—without a second thought.

The Proof Is Here

When the Body Moves Correctly, the Body Heals

By learning how to tap into your natural healing power you'll be doing one of the best things you've ever done for yourself. Employing the Core Program, I've seen amazing, life-altering changes over and over again.

Laura, at 36, came to see me because of unrelenting arm, wrist and hand pain. "It's carpal tunnel syndrome," she stated emphatically. "I work all day at the computer and I've had X rays and an electromyogram. The tests didn't pinpoint any obvious physical problem, and medication didn't help. I was told that wrist surgery might help—but I'm not crazy about that idea."

My examination revealed that Laura's problem was not in her wrist, but rather in her neck. There, a shortening of nerve roots in her cervical spine, caused by poor posture and weak back muscles, was triggering her pain. Treating her neck with core exercises made Laura's hand problem disappear in a matter of days.

Roz figured that the source of her sore back was an old mattress, but replacing it with an extra-firm variety didn't make her feel any better. "I've increased my upper-body workouts on the machines at my health club but my back feels worse. Not only that, I'm so stiff that when I bend forward my fingertips barely reach midshins—never mind my toes. I'm only 34—am I going to end up totally disabled?"

I could see that the muscles in the back of Roz's thighs and lower back were abnormally shortened. Using my Core Program gave her much-needed relief in less than a week. Less than two months later, her back pain was nothing but a distant memory.

Christy, an avid exerciser, complained to her doctor during a yearly checkup about her increasingly painful knees. She resented it when he brushed off her concern with a comment about how, at 41, she wasn't a kid anymore and she should expect her knees to feel sore. "I dread the thought of increased deterioration as I age. I love to ski and I'm really distressed about having to give it up," she explained. When, after thoroughly examining her, I pointed out that her concerns were real but very treatable, she shouted with joy. Two months after beginning the Core Program exercises, Christy was able to jog three miles with no discomfort. Today she tells me she feels better than she did in her twenties.

Jessica was just 32 when she first wrenched her back picking up her three-year-old son. "I figured that lower-back pain went hand-in-hand with raising a child," she told me. "But when I lifted a bag of cat litter and felt what could only be described as agony, I knew something was really wrong. I tried bed rest, yoga and a variety of over-the-counter painkillers, but nothing worked," she told me as she rubbed her ever-aching back.

When I told her to lie on her stomach and arch backward she smiled gratefully. This exercise virtually eliminated her pain by stretching the lower back and relieving pressure on compressed nerves. Jessica knew she could perform it at home to optimize her healing on a daily basis. Indeed, she found much-needed relief within days. She was then ready for my Core Program. After two months of daily exercise, Jessica fully regained the strength in her back. Now, keeping up with her active little boy is a pleasure.

THE BEST MAKEOVER YOU'LL EVER HAVE

With the Core Program, you, like Laura, Roz, Christy and Jessica, are going to get a terrific makeover—and this one will last a lifetime. My regimen *will* heal what is off-balance in your body because I don't treat symptoms of dysfunction. Instead, *I treat the problem at its core.*

SPECIAL CORE, SPECIAL NEEDS

Through my training, observation and hands-on experience, as well as through facing my own physical obstacles, I know that the physical and lifestyle cores of women affect seven particular areas—I call them "hot spots"—that require special attention.

Cooling the "hot spots"—and preventing them from heating up again—is one of the major objectives of the Core Program. The "hot spots" I focus on are the following:

- neck
- shoulder complex, which includes the upper back
- abdominal zone
- lower back
- pelvic area
- hips
- lower extremities, which include the knees, ankles and feet

Take These Self-Tests

There's a simple way to determine if any of your "hot spots" are heating up. Each test reveals any imbalances you might have. Please don't worry if you don't "pass" one or more of the tests. The point of taking them is to give you important information about your body. Remember too that one imbalance is often connected to another, which is why you may have difficulty with more than one test. For instance, neck pain is often associated with the back, and knee pain is linked to the hips or feet.

Once you pinpoint your hot spots, you have the power to cool them by doing the Core Program. And the Core Program exercises will also prevent them from flaring up again.

The self-tests have one more function. Use them to assess the changes you are making in your body. After doing the Core Program for three weeks, take the tests again—and be amazed at the difference.

After you do each test, check the appropriate response.

**FOR HOT SPOT #1, THE NECK,
TAKE THIS NECK ROTATION TEST.**
Sit down and look straight ahead. Then slowly turn your head as far as you can to the right and then to the left, with your chin aligned with your shoulder.

Next, keep your upper back erect and lower your chin so that it touches your chest.

Finally, lift your head up again and stretch backward until your face is parallel to the ceiling.

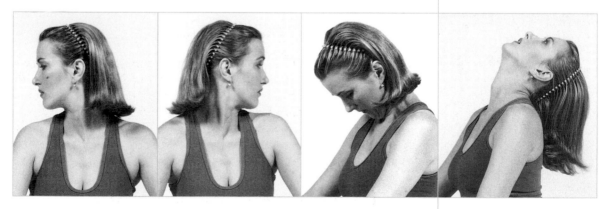

5. Extremely difficult
4. Very difficult
3. Difficult
2. Slightly difficult
1. Not difficult

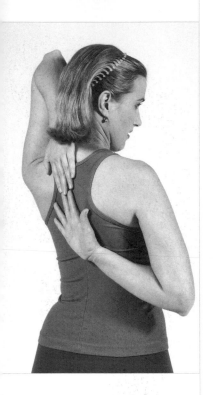

If you experience difficulty moving in any direction, your neck muscles, as well as your shoulder muscles, may have become shortened.

FOR HOT SPOT #2, THE SHOULDER COMPLEX (AND UPPER BACK), TAKE THIS SHOULDER MOTION TEST.

Stand up. Raise your left arm overhead and bend it behind you with your palm on your upper back, letting that hand dangle down your back as far as possible. Rotate your right arm behind your waist and try to reach up and grab your left hand with your right. Then reverse arms.

    5. Extremely difficult
    4. Very difficult
    3. Difficult
    2. Slightly difficult
    1. Not difficult

If you have any discomfort doing this, it shows that your shoulder muscles are extremely tight. If it's easier to do the test on one side than the other, it means that there is an imbalance between the muscles on the right and left sides of your body.

FOR HOT SPOT #3, THE ABDOMINAL ZONE, TAKE THIS ABDOMINAL STRENGTH TEST.

Lie on your back with your arms at your sides. Raise your head, neck and shoulders off the floor (as if you were doing a sit-up) and lift your arms with the palms up. At the same time lift your legs up several inches with heels pressed together and toes pointing outward. Hold for thirty seconds.

    5. Extremely difficult
    4. Very difficult
    3. Difficult
    2. Slightly difficult
    1. Not difficult

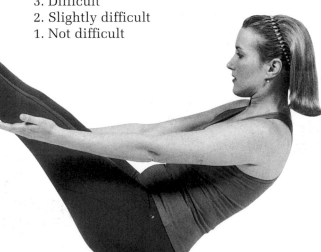

If you can't do this or have trouble maintaining the position for thirty seconds, it shows that your abdominal muscles, along with your inner thigh and hip muscles, are not as strong as they could be.

FOR HOT SPOT #4, THE LOWER BACK, TAKE THESE RANGE OF MOTION TESTS.

a) Standing erect, with feet shoulder-width apart, bend over with straight legs and touch your toes.

Roll up to standing, press your palms to your buttocks and bend backward. Exhale as your chest lifts toward the ceiling and continue to tilt your head backward. Return to the starting position.

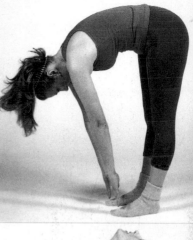

5. Extremely difficult
4. Very difficult
3. Difficult
2. Slightly difficult
1. Not difficult

b) Lie on your back with your arms at your sides.

Without arching your back, tighten your thigh and pull your left leg straight back, toward your torso, to a 90 degree angle. Don't lift or bend your right leg. Put your left leg down and repeat test with the right leg.

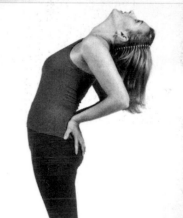

5. Extremely difficult
4. Very difficult
3. Difficult
2. Slightly difficult
1. Not difficult

If you can't do these movements, it means that your lower-back muscles are tight, as are your hamstring muscles, which help extend your hips and flex your knees. The hamstrings also work to control your pelvis and your spine. Additionally, your abdominals may not be strong enough to stabilize your pelvis, which makes it difficult to hold your leg straight up.

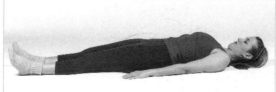

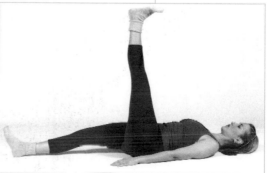

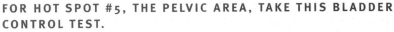

FOR HOT SPOT #5, THE PELVIC AREA, TAKE THIS BLADDER CONTROL TEST.

To test the strength of the muscles that support your bladder and urethra, consciously stop your urine stream for three seconds while you are sitting on the toilet.

(Please do not do this as an exercise! Doing so will give you a dysfunctional bladder.)

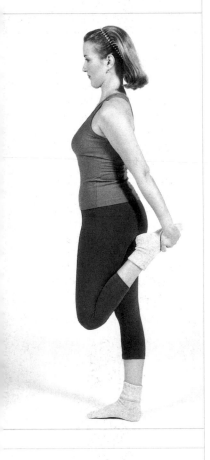

5. Extremely difficult
4. Very difficult
3. Difficult
2. Slightly difficult
1. Not difficult

If you can't do this, it shows that your pelvic muscles aren't as strong as they could be. (If you have been doing Kegel exercises, you have been doing them incorrectly. See page 67.)

FOR HOT SPOT #6, THE HIPS, TAKE THIS FRONT THIGH TEST.

While balanced on the right foot, bend and lift your left leg behind you, grabbing your left foot in your left hand. Bend your knee until the foot reaches your buttock without arching your back. For balance, extend your right arm in front of you. Repeat this test with your right leg.

5. Extremely difficult
4. Very difficult
3. Difficult
2. Slightly difficult
1. Not difficult

If you can't do the test on one or both legs it means that both hip flexors, the muscles that stabilize the pelvis when you move your legs, and your thigh muscles are tight.

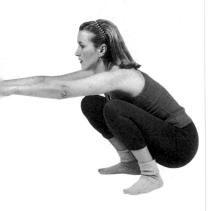

FOR HOT SPOT #7, THE LOWER EXTREMITIES, TAKE THIS DEEP SQUAT TEST.

Stand up with your feet shoulder-width apart. Now squat down with your heels flat on the floor with your buttocks resting on your heels. Don't let your feet roll inward. Keep your kneecaps aligned over your second toes. Reach your arms straight out in front of you.

5. Extremely difficult
4. Very difficult
3. Difficult
2. Slightly difficult
1. Not difficult

If you can't do this easily, it means that your ankles are tight, your hips lack flexibility and the hamstring muscles may be shortened. Also, your knees don't have a full range of motion.

And now for one last test. The balance test reveals the power and strength of all the muscles in your lower extremities. This doesn't address any of the hot spots, but balance is important in everything you do. And strong core muscles contribute a lot of your ability to balance by stabilizing your pelvis.

HOW DID YOU DO?

Did you "pass" the tests with flying colors? If so, you're one of the very few people who do. Even professional athletes tend to lack strength or flexibility in some of the muscle groups. In fact, I don't think there's anyone who wouldn't benefit from doing the Core Program exercises, all of which are designed to balance and strengthen the muscles that give us so much trouble in our "hot spot" areas. For those of you who are already "strong at the core," use these exercises to make sure you stay that way.

Check Your Balance

Put a piece of paper on the floor as your mark. Standing on one foot, jump up and down on that paper ten times, landing with slightly bent knee. Switch to your opposite foot and repeat.

If you have trouble completing this exercise, or you continually miss the paper, your balance is not as good as it could be. Balance requires the power of foot and ankle strength and motor control (the ability to slowly elongate muscles for deceleration as you use them) as well as abdominal and overall leg strength.

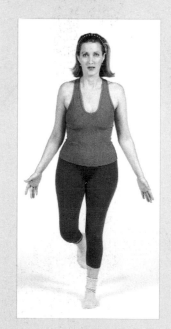

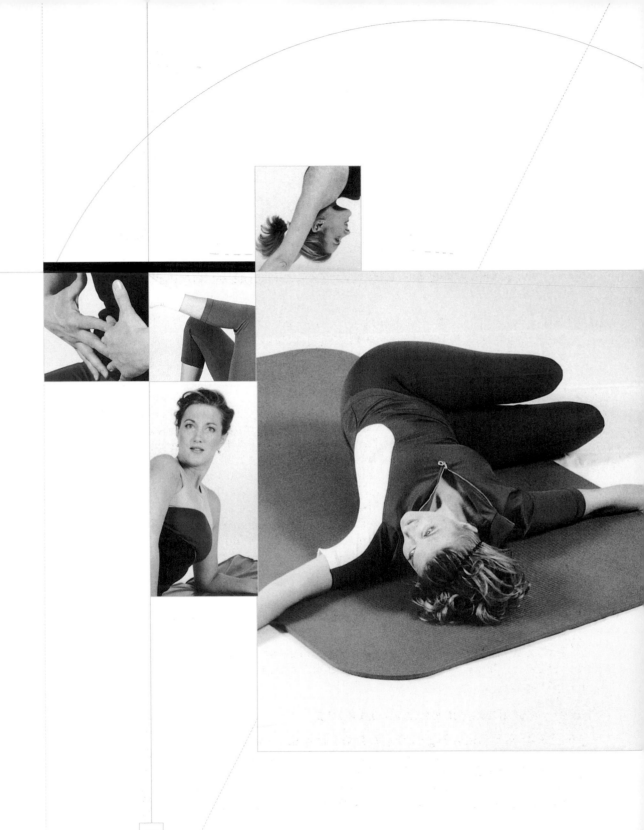

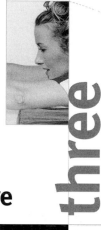

my journey to the core

Before I could help other women, I had to learn to help myself. Discovering how my own body worked was the beginning of a life-long pursuit. My journey of discovery began very early and continues to this day.

FIRST IMPRESSION

When a patient asks me why I became a physical therapist instead of a doctor, I tell her that I love the hands-on work I do. I also talk about the profound influence of my grandmother.

By the time I was seven she had lost both her legs to diabetes and was living in a nursing home. I used to visit her as often as I could. Overweight and weak, and suffering from severe diabetes, my grandmother lived the last years of her life in a wheelchair. Around her sat unmoving men and women, too feeble to lift a spoon, with catheters attached to their bladders. It was a scene that was profoundly unnerving and depressing. Often I would say to my mother when we left, "This isn't right. Why do people have to end up like this?"

"I don't know," my mother would reply. "All I do know is that Grammie thinks what happened to her couldn't be avoided."

But I couldn't accept that. Even as a child I somehow knew this couldn't be right. I was intuitively certain that such things *could* be avoided.

MY OWN HEALTH CRISIS BEGINS

Until I started junior high school, I was just like the other neighborhood kids in northern New Jersey. I rode my bicycle to school, played with my friends and lived the typical suburban life.

However, while dealing with the usual awkwardness of puberty, I also began to suffer some problems that seemed particularly my own. Trembling hands and bulging eyes were the start. Then my appetite became insatiable as my weight plummeted and eczema blotched my skin with scaly dry spots. My concentration in school fell.

One morning I awoke with a severely swollen neck. My mother immediately called our family pediatrician for a consultation. After seeing him I was referred to a well-respected endocrinologist for emergency care because it had been determined that I had a hyperactive thyroid that was dangerously out of control. My blood pressure was so high and my heart rate so elevated that I was actually at risk for a stroke or a heart attack.

The specialist diagnosed hyperthyroidism, also known as Graves' disease, which meant that my thyroid gland had gone into overdrive and was pumping out way too much of the hormone thyroxin. Consequently, my entire system was thrown off-kilter. The hormone produced by the thyroid, he explained, was responsible for all electrical and chemical reactions in the body. It also played an important role in regulating the body's metabolic rate. My thyroid problem, he went on, explained my extreme thinness; people with thyroid disorders are prone to either gain or lose a significant amount of weight.

While he gave me medications that helped me, he didn't offer any guidance for living a healthy life. After two years of taking prescription drugs that saved my life, I was told by the endocrinologist that my condition had not adequately improved. There was only one thing he could now recommend and his proposal was truly alarming. He suggested the surgical removal of my thyroid gland. But that wasn't going to be the end of it. I'd have to take replacement thyroid hormone in pill form for the rest of my life. Then there was even more bad news. Complications, such as infertility, depression and obesity, might develop years after the surgery.

I became enraged. Only fifteen years old, I already had plenty to deal with and was not prepared to handle more bad news. The drug I'd been given to slow down my out-of-control thyroid had significantly slowed down my metabolism as well. I was carrying around forty extra pounds, which not only made me extremely uncomfortable but also made me the target of more than a few cruel comments from my classmates. Now I was imagining myself becoming even heavier. But even worse was that the surgery would involve cutting my neck open, which would leave a visible scar. I'd have yet another "mark" to add to the long list of physical abnormalities that were the result of my condition. I was absolutely determined not to have the recommended surgery.

My mother, thankfully, was always open to finding different ways to approach a problem—and she did!

THE FIRST ALTERNATIVE

My mother found a doctor (an M.D. who also had a Ph.D.) at a nearby medical research center who was starting a thyroid study using megavitamin therapy to reverse hyperthyroidism. After I was accepted in the study, I was given nearly two dozen different vitamins to take every day over the next year and a half.

The treatment started to work, but being a typical teenager I began to resent having to take so many pills. When, after six months on this regimen, the first thyroid test results came back normal, I decided to stop taking the capsules. I chose to ignore the doctor who had advised me that, by the end of the next twelve months, the vitamins would probably be able to restore my thyroid to completely normal function for the rest of my life and I would be able to stop taking them.

Not yet sixteen and finally feeling healthy again, I was convinced my body would maintain its newfound vigor. Why continue with the regimen? I was sure I was cured.

I was wrong. Within six weeks, my thyroid problems returned full blown. I didn't know what to do.

A NEW STRATEGY

Once again my mother helped me find a way out of my problem. She took me to visit an alternative-medicine practitioner, a body healer named Margabandhu. My mother believed in Margabandhu because his use of acupressure and therapeutic massage, along with dietary changes, had helped a close friend of hers overcome a severe digestive disorder.

"You have an imbalance in your endocrine system caused by energy blocked in your neck," he told me. "I'm trying to get the energy, or chi, as it is referred to in Eastern medicine, flowing again in order to get your body back into a balanced state."

Listening to Margabandhu, I felt something new. For the first time someone was giving me hope that I could return to a naturally healthy state, and that I could do that without the help of an intense medical regimen involving prescription medications, surgery or massive doses of vitamins.

Instead, with Margabandhu's guidance, I was going to learn how to tap into the power of self-healing. As he worked on my body to restore its balance, Margabandhu taught me the laws of health—diet, sleep, exercise, relaxation.

THE ALTERNATIVE THAT WORKED

I went to Margabandhu every week for the next year, and my mother made sure that I returned to doctors at regular intervals to check my thyroxin levels. At the end of the year the levels were completely within normal limits.

I not only looked much better, I felt terrific. I knew that Margabandhu had given me the tools to keep myself healthy. I didn't feel like a guinea pig, the way I had with the vitamin study. Instead I felt that I was learning to tune in to my body. When I cheated a bit, and ate some things I wasn't supposed to, I didn't feel well. That was an immediate and clear lesson in cause and effect, and I found it fascinating.

Margabandhu was such an inspiration to me that I became his student. In between college classes, I regularly traveled to his busy office to study massage therapy, yoga and meditation. Working closely with him, I observed the people he was able to aid after mainstream doctors lost interest in them. He helped relieve allergies in longtime hay fever sufferers, alleviate attention deficit disorder in school-age children and resolve musculoskeletal problems in office workers.

After more than a year of intensive training with Margabandhu, I became a certified massage therapist and soon after that started my own business working solely with women. Listening to them as I kneaded their muscles, I heard what was to become a familiar litany of discomforts. Many of the clients complained of aching backs, stiff joints and bothersome necks, even though many were still in their thirties or even younger. More than a few women confessed that they didn't feel as good as they thought they should, but believed there was nothing they could do about it.

What they said made a big impression on me. I began to read everything I could find on healing the body through manipulation.

SEEKING MY OWN ANSWERS

For a long time I had considered going to medical school, but when I weighed the differences between how traditional medicine approached physical problems and how alternative practitioners dealt with them, I changed my mind.

While I had enormous regard for much of the lifesaving work done by doctors—and I still do—I strongly believed that my own particular area of concentration should not be centered solely on traditional medicine. In my experience, Western medicine treated the symptoms while excluding the whole person, which meant it could never get to the core of the problem. The solutions it offered always seemed to come from the outside, and often they were either drastic in nature, such as surgery, or experimental, such as the megavitamin study I had been in. None of them harnessed the power of the body to heal itself, and that's what I wanted to learn to do.

Still, the more I was pulled toward understanding the inner workings of the body, the more I realized that Western medicine had to be part of my education. Massage therapy, which didn't include any pathology training, didn't teach me how to address the problems of a specific body area with precision. Additionally, I wanted to show people how to keep their bodies in tip-top condition and fight off infirmity. To do that, I knew I needed science-based clinical training.

I didn't know what area of health care would take me to the juncture where traditional and alternative medicine meet. Margabandhu, yet again, came to my rescue. He pointed out that physical therapy involved medical science and tapped into the ability of the body to heal itself when it moved correctly.

THE PHYSICAL THERAPY APPROACH

One of the most compelling aspects of physical therapy is the wide range of medical problems on which it has an impact. Patients who are grappling with orthopedic injuries, sports-related injuries, brain trauma, women's health issues and spinal rehabilitation—and even cardiopulmonary illnesses—can all benefit enormously from physical therapy. That's because the aim of the physical ther-

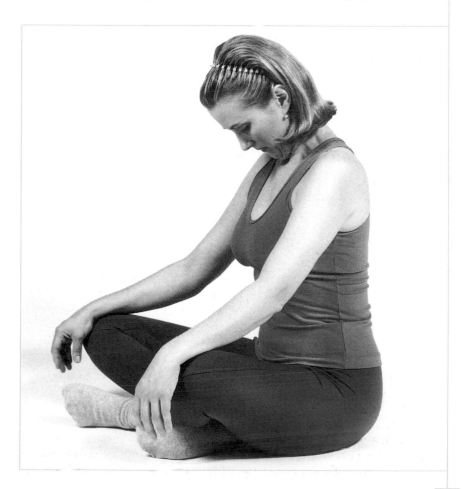

apist is to help patients move and feel better, no matter what their overall condition is. The field includes an extensive study of human anatomy, physiology, pathology, physics, chemistry, motor learning and motor control.

Each physical therapy patient is assessed not only to treat her musculoskeletal symptoms, but also to correct the underlying cause of her decreased function. Therapists screen and treat problems stemming from postural imbalance, muscular weakness or abnormal joint mobility, each of which can lead to further injury. Physical therapy also includes an important preventive aspect. If a patient has experienced injuries, learning to move correctly as well as how to strengthen and balance her body will help prevent recurrences.

As I studied physical therapy, I began to develop an increased awareness of my own body that really took me by surprise. For example, I had always taken for granted the fact that, ever since I was a teenager, I could not lie on my stomach without feeling back pain. And, right after getting up, I couldn't move around easily. Once I started doing certain stretches, those problems ended. I also learned how to deal with much more serious problems in my body.

Over the course of the next few years, I found that I could self-treat tendinitis, and I healed myself of several herniated disks in my neck and lower back. While in college, I suffered whiplash neck injuries from two minor car accidents and each time I found I knew what to do to alleviate my discomfort.

Ironically enough, I even had to use my newfound knowledge of physical therapy to relieve the bad effects of the incredibly long hours I spent sitting in chairs that gave me poor support in my physical therapy classes! By the time I was twenty-three, I suffered frequent episodes of daily neck and lower-back pain, just like those women who came to me for treatment. Now, however, I knew what movements to do to give myself relief.

My first job as a physical therapist was at the John F. Kennedy Medical Center in New Jersey. Originally, I was assigned to outpatient orthopedics and the chronic pain clinic. There I saw that the best results came from educating patients to do exercises that got their bodies moving correctly. My second rotation was working in acute care, which covered the postoperative, oncology and pediatric units. I saw immediately how patients improved when their muscles received specific exercises. My last hospital rotation was practicing physical therapy in the brain-trauma unit, where I treated severely head-injured patients. It was there that I saw more clearly than ever how the body's ability to heal can be enhanced through proper intervention and facilitated movement.

THE CORE OF MY PRACTICE

By the time I opened my physical therapy practice a short time later, I had decided to concentrate on the musculoskeletal problems of women. As I listened to my female patients telling me about their lifestyles, I began to see how certain behaviors impacted on their bodies. At the same time, I kept studying to learn all I could about how the structure of the female body affected the musculoskeletal system. What I was learning seemed relevant to everything from urinary stress incontinence to osteoporosis, from the strength and muscle deficiencies of postmastectomy patients to the minor but debilitating discomforts of women who sat at a computer screen all day.

Whenever I treated a patient, I would give her three exercises for her injuries. Then I would observe what was working, and add or take away exercises as needed in the days that followed. I monitored what she was doing and kept precise medical notes of what worked. Over and over again I saw that when the core moved as it should, the body could heal itself. The Core Program was the outcome, and the results were phenomenal!

My experience during these years showed me that the purpose of my work was to empower others with knowledge about their bodies. I could give them exercises to enhance their resilience against disease and aging and restore the quality of their daily lives. The dream of being healthy could become real.

At last, I had found the core of my professional life.

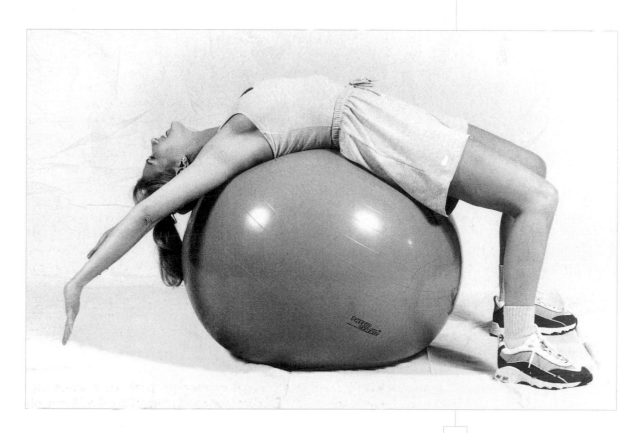

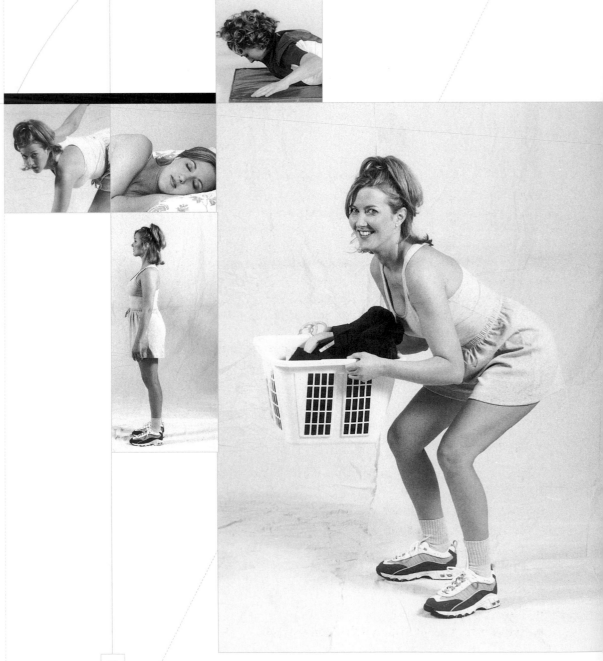

gracious against gravity

GRAVITY: THE FORCE THAT IS WITH YOU

When I ask a patient how she thinks gravity affects her, she usually raises her eyebrows, frowns and quickly points to either her breasts or her buttocks. Sometimes she places her hands on either side of her face and pulls the skin back in a mock attempt at a face-lift.

Instead of viewing gravity as the enemy, it's time to reestablish a good working relationship with this monumental force. Gravity can be one of your best allies, because how you hold your body against gravity can improve your strength and prevent osteoporosis. Good posture maximizes respiratory capacity, which means you breathe more deeply. This, in turn, lessens fatigue. When the bond between you and the earth's pull is as nature intended it to be, you will reap these benefits—and you will feel great.

However, if there are problems in your relationship, you'll know it. I call the indicators of these problems red flags.

THE RED FLAGS

There are a number of clear indicators of a relationship with gravity gone wrong. They include:

- Feeling stiff in the morning
- Difficulty in getting out of bed
- Painful heels
- Pain or strain when lifting
- General achiness
- Creaking joints
- Fatigue, no matter how much sleep you get

Here's an easy self-test that will show you how sitting upright gives you maximum strength. You can test yourself, but if you don't trust the results ask a friend to help you.

Slouch in a chair and put your writing hand on a table with the pinkie side of your hand facing down and your thumb toward the ceiling. Put gentle pressure against your thumb as you try to prevent it from being pushed toward the table. What happens?

Now, sit up straight, with your lower back pressed into the back of the chair, and repeat the test. What happens this time?

When you sit upright your fingers receive the maximum nerve firings to your muscles which, in turn, give you the strength you need. Slouching, on the other hand, cuts off the nerve impulses and leaves you weak. So remember: Sit tall and stay strong.

In my experience, these symptoms can often be traced to a failure to position the body against gravity in the most effective way. Whether you are sitting or standing or moving, your muscles need to be balanced and your joints need to be in alignment, so that your body exerts an upward force equal in intensity to the gravity that pulls you downward. Only if you are strong, straight down to the core, can you achieve that kind of balance and alignment.

WHY YOU FEEL TIRED

If you get eight hours of sleep a night and eat a nutritious diet and still feel tired during the day, it may be due to your posture.

When you do a job and don't receive the postural support you need, you have to work harder to get the job done. The extra effort tires you out. Your muscles are the same way. When they work at a disadvantage they must work harder against gravity, and not surprisingly, they fatigue more easily.

Here's an example. If, like so many of us, you sit at a computer for hours every day, you may find yourself slouching. When that happens the pectoral muscles in your chest shorten. Blood vessels that supply the muscles with oxygen and nutrients, along with the nerves that fire electrical impulses to the muscles, get compressed. At the same time, the muscles in your back lengthen and weaken.

Gravity is going to keep pulling you forward, further shortening the pectoral muscles. The joints that are supported and held in place by these muscles are going to be pulled out of alignment. Consequently, holding yourself upright is going to be harder to do and you are going to feel tired.

There are other effects as well. Not maintaining a properly aligned upright position can hamper the functioning of your vital organs. Slumping compresses the abdomen, which restricts peristalsis, the wavelike muscular contractions that push food through your intestines for absorption and elimination. Slumping also restricts the movement of the lungs and impedes breathing and digestion. When your chest is pulled down, breathing becomes shallow instead of deep. Your head slants forward, which affects proper blood flow to the brain. Not surprisingly, you will feel sluggish and begin to lose mental sharpness.

You may not realize it, but your head weighs between ten and twelve pounds—the weight of a bowling ball. When your head is not in the neutral position, that is, held straight up from the neck, a sequence of events begins to unfold. Compressed disks in the neck interrupt the firing of nerve cells in the lower neck, the arms and the hands. Pain and weakness strike, resulting in headaches, jaw tension, shoulder problems and overall discomfort. (See chapter five, page 59, for injuries stemming from the neck "hot spot.")

USE GRAVITY TO YOUR ADVANTAGE

The Core Program draws you up and out from your core, counteracting the force of gravity, which pulls you down and in. The core exercises reestablish a positive relationship with gravitational forces, allowing you to increase your strength, circulation and well-being.

The exercises follow the basics of neurological development by moving muscles the way you developed them in order to sit up, stand and walk.

Think of what a baby does. Lying on her belly, she first learns to raise her head and then begins to turn it from side to side. Then, having developed enough strength to support her head, her torso begins to arch away from the surface she's lying on so that her chest and her legs can rise a few inches, and her hands and feet, too. Lifting her torso against the force of gravity in this way develops the strength she will need to be able to sit up by herself, which most babies do at around six months. And this is why I have included in each of the Core programs one version or another of an exercise called the Butterfly, which works on the same principles—mobilizing your back and stomach muscles to keep you stable as you lift up your torso against gravity. Your entire spine is strengthened in the process.

BE LONG AND STRONG

"I've been self-conscious about being large-chested since I was a teenager, and I always hunched over," Stephanie, a 29-year-old who complained of constant fatigue, told me. "Doing the Core Program helped me a lot. I started to feel strength in my back right away, which made it easier to stand, and sit, straight. Not only that—I've started to feel a lot more energized."

The Core Program works the front and back muscles of the torso, the muscles that hold you up. Strengthening them enables you to sit or stand straight up for longer periods of time, which in turn minimizes the wear and tear on your joints. By repositioning your body, you will restore the normal alignment of your joints from head to toe. With proper alignment comes added energy, since all the muscles, and the nerves within them, are working at maximum efficiency.

Strong core muscles make your body capable of maintaining perfect posture all the time. No matter what you are doing—sitting, rising, standing, walking, squatting or even sleeping—your muscles will allow your joints to move efficiently.

Even before you begin the Core Program, you can begin to align yourself when you sit, lift or even sleep. Here's how.

Don't Get Out of Joint

If you awaken stiff and achy you are feeling the effect of muscle tension, which is causing the joints to go out of alignment. For example, if your shoulder is tense you won't sleep in a relaxed position. Instead, you'll get yourself into a position that further shortens the shoulder muscle and compresses the shoulder joint. When you awaken, that shoulder will feel stiff. Here's a tip: Do the Head-to-Toe Prep, the first exercise of the Core Foundation, before you go to sleep. It releases muscle tension so your body stays in neutral alignment. You'll awake feeling rested and pain-free.

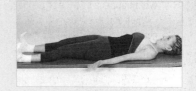

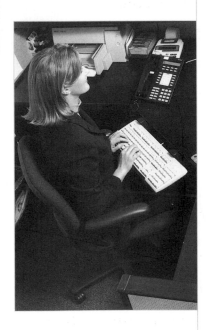

Using a lumbar roll will support the lower back. (You can also use a rolled-up towel.)

SIT DOWN AND MAKE YOURSELF COMFORTABLE

So many women must sit for a long part of their day, which is the best reason I know to be both comfortable and aligned.

- Be sure to choose a good ergonomically designed work chair with adjustable height and armrests and a tilting backrest. Your entire upper body should be either upright or tilted forward slightly. Use a small pillow or towel roll to support your lower back. (And do the same thing when you're at home, whether you are working or relaxing.)
- Keep your shoulders back and straight.
- Elbows should be close to your sides, bent at a 90 degree angle instead of extended out in front of your body. (Never let your forearms rest on the desk's sharp edge. This puts too much pressure on sensitive superficial nerves that can easily be damaged.)
- Knees are either the same level with, or slightly below, your hips.
- Feet are either flat on the floor or supported on a footrest slightly out in front of the knees (especially if you are wearing heels).
- Place the computer monitor at arm's length and at eye level. If you are right-handed, put the phone on the left of the desk and the mouse on the right (vice versa if you are left-handed), both within close reach. I also advise using a headset. This practical device will prevent you from clamping the receiver between your ear and shoulder, which strains your neck.
- Keep your head straight or with the chin tilted slightly downward. Place whatever you need to read at eye level to eliminate the need to constantly turn and bend your head while you type. There are many devices that hold papers at the right height, including one that attaches to a computer monitor.
- As you work, relax your wrists in a slightly angled upward position. This prevents nerves from being compressed between bones and tendons, which contributes to carpal tunnel syndrome.
- Change your position frequently. Even if your chair and desk are adjusted perfectly, shift your position at least every hour or so to prevent muscle fatigue and encourage circulation in your spine.
- To rise, slide forward to the edge of the chair. Pivot forward from your hips and use your leg muscles to stand up.

"I caught myself slouching at my desk because it felt more comfortable that way. At the same time, the back and sides of my neck always felt strained," Elaine, 34 years old, told me. "After I started the Core Program I felt better sitting up, and the tension in my neck disappeared."

Elaine needed a way to strengthen her torso to counter-

act the effects of slouching. Exercising the muscles in the upper and lower abdomen, as well as the muscles of the back and buttocks, made sitting straight easier. At the same time she alleviated a nagging neck strain.

GET A GOOD NIGHT'S SLEEP

The hours you spend in sleep allow your body to restore itself. Make the most of that time by sleeping in a position that maximizes comfort and minimizes strain on your most vulnerable muscles. For example, don't sleep on your stomach. Doing so makes your lower back sag, which will increase pressure on your back. Also, it's not good for your neck, and it may limit blood supply to your brain by as much as 40 percent.

Your pillow should be wide enough to avoid any head tilting when you lie on your side. I suggest using an extra pillow in one of two ways.

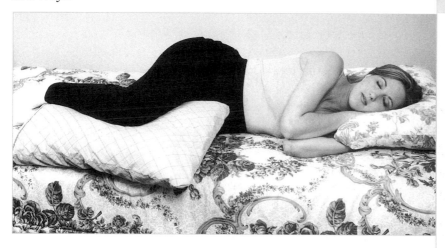

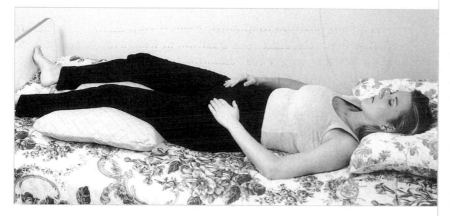

When you sleep on your side, place a pillow between your knees to keep your spine and pelvis in an aligned position throughout the night. You'll avoid nerve impingements and muscle strains.

When you rest on your back, place a pillow under your knees. Using a pillow this way, especially if your lower back is sore, offers wonderful—albeit temporary—decompression of the vertebral joints and disks. Don't, however, sleep a full night in this position. If you do, the soft tissue that encases the nerve roots throughout the lower spine will shorten, thereby narrowing the openings by which the nerves exit the spinal cord. This adaptive shortening makes assuming an upright position more difficult. And it may contribute to the bent-over posture seen in some elderly people.

CARRYING THE LOAD

While you might not be doing the kind of job that requires continuous lifting, it is inevitable that you'll have to bend and pick up a few things throughout your day. Here's how to do it to prevent injury.

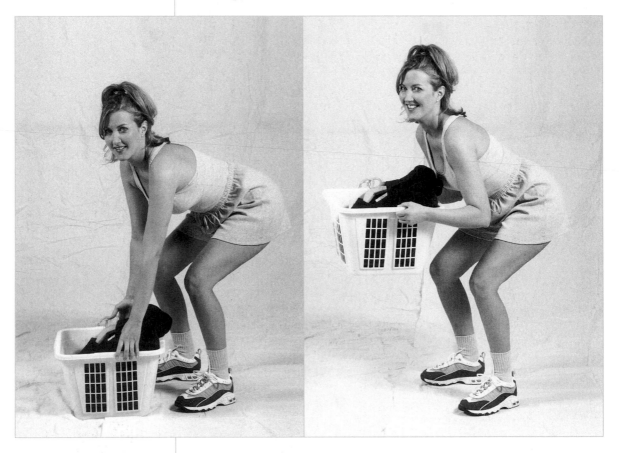

- Start with a solid base of support with your feet flat on the ground, shoulder-width apart.

- Keep your upper back straight and your lower back in the neutral position. Don't bend forward from the waist to lift.

- Bend your knees as if you're squatting over a public toilet, and let your strong gluteals and legs do the work instead of your back. Tighten your abdominal muscles and buttocks to further support your back.

- Keep the load as close to your body as possible.

- When shifting a heavy object, turn your whole body by pivoting on your feet to avoid twisting your back.

- Never lift a heavy object higher than shoulder level. If you need to hoist it higher, use a footstool or a ladder.

A GREAT REASON TO REALIGN YOUR SPINE

After years of professional experience and clinical observation, I can emphatically state that proper spinal alignment against gravity helps prevent osteoporosis.

When the spine is aligned as it should be, each vertebra is stacked one on top of the other following the natural curves of the spine. Think of a stack of tripods to envision how these bones connect. Each vertebra touches the next one at three points. At the rear of each vertebra is a pair of bony protrusions called the facets, which form two contact points. The third contact point is the disk at the front of each vertebra. When all three points connect, each vertebra is bearing the weight of its neighbor in a cascading effect that promotes the formation of new bone cells.

If, however, all three points do not connect because spinal alignment is off, the weight-bearing effect will be lost. Bones won't regenerate and will, inevitably, become brittle.

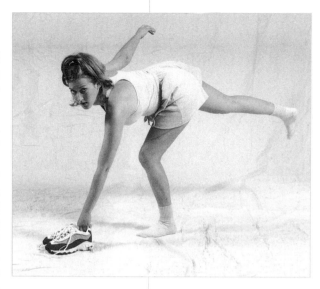

Golfer's lift. You should lift a small object—like a sneaker—the way a golfer does, with one leg off the ground.

TRAIN YOUR BONES TO GROW

The Core Program is a proven, efficient system to build bone where your body needs it.

First, the Core Program allows maximal weight bearing through the spine and the bones of the lower forearm to the wrist, and the

Lifting a child. Here's the right way to lift and carry a child. First, face the child and bring her close. Next, use your legs and buttocks to lift her up.

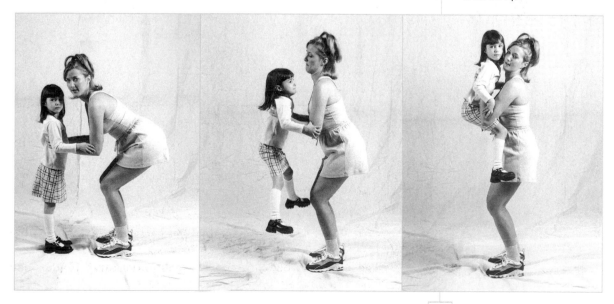

upper thigh to the hip, to prompt the creation of bone cells at the most common sites of osteoporosis.

Second, the exercises use body weight as a resistive force against gravity, which also helps to build bone mass.

Third, the core exercises make sure that opposing muscles pull equally on bones. To do this, muscles that are either too shortened or too lengthened are restored to their proper length. With muscle balance restored and the joints now in alignment, the equal tug on bone stimulates the creation of new bone cells. In short, by doing these exercises you will have created an efficient system to replenish bone mass where it is needed.

> *After Paula, 45, fell on an icy street and shattered her wrist, she came to see me and immediately voiced her concerns. "As soon as my wrist broke I thought about my mother and her sister. Both of them have osteoporosis. I'm worried about getting it, too."*
>
> *Whether or not her broken wrist could be attributed to early osteoporosis, I had no way of knowing at that moment. What I did know was that I could give Paula some protection against it with appropriate exercise. Once Paula began doing the Core Program she began to increase the muscle power in her upper body through exercises that strengthen the upper and lower muscles of the back, and also the muscles that pull the shoulder blades closer to the spine. This helped align her shoulders, and allowed the muscles within to work more effectively. And, once her wrist was healed, she was eventually able to move on to the Ultimate Core Program, which includes exercises that boost arm power through the use of hand weights.*
>
> *In addition, she was stretching the tissues of the upper body, including the pectoral muscles, which tend to shorten through daily activity, and relieving tension on the nerves that traverse the shoulders and the lower portion of the neck and upper back. The Butterfly exercise in all three Core Programs, as well as the Advanced Mermaid in the Ultimate Core, helped her build up her neck muscles to give her head better support.*

OSTEOPOROSIS: IT'S NOT INEVITABLE

By the turn of the millennium, more than 26 million Americans had been diagnosed with osteoporosis, which is defined as a bone density that is 25 percent or more below the peak bone mass for your age. More than three quarters of those diagnosed with osteoporosis were women.

Women lose bone density because of a number of factors. The decline in estrogen that occurs after menopause is a key factor but by no means the only one. Smoking, drinking excessive amounts of alcohol and downing sodas like colas that contain phosphoric acid—all leach calcium from the bones. Certain drugs prescribed for inflammation, including hydrocortisone, cortisone, prednisone and prednisolone can also cause bone loss. A calcium-deficient diet, along with lack of physical activity, also contributes to the weakening of the bones.

Having seen how osteoporosis contributes to the suffering I encounter among the women in my practice, I am very determined to do what I can to help prevent this degenerative disease. Its symptoms include:

- a constant dull ache in a hip, or a pain that fans out across the shoulder blades or middle back. But, unlike typical muscle aches, the pain of osteoporosis doesn't diminish with either time, rest or medication.

- bone breaks stemming from everyday behaviors like bending over to pick up a newspaper, stepping off a curb, getting a hug or sneezing.

- the inability to walk unassisted, or to summon the strength to open a window.

- changes in appearance that have serious consequences far beyond any cosmetic concerns. As vertebrae at the top of the neck slide forward, the spine curves and eventually creates the back deformity known as dowager's hump. Then, as lower ribs close in on the upper abdomen, the midsection narrows and the abdomen protrudes. Lung capacity is severely reduced in the process.

You *can* stop the onset and progression of this terrible disease. Fifteen minutes a day is all it takes to keep you straight and strong. And remember that proper calcium intake is critical: Exercise puts a demand on bones to increase osteoblasts, the bone-forming cells that require calcium. That means 1,000 milligrams a day up to the onset of menopause, and 1,500 milligrams a day thereafter. Since most of us don't get enough calcium from the food we eat, taking calcium supplements will ensure that you get what you need.

HOW DO YOU STACK UP?

I give this alignment assessment test to all my patients. Stand in front of a full-length mirror. Keep your arms relaxed at your sides with your feet shoulder-width apart.

YOU HAVE PROPER ALIGNMENT IF YOUR:

- Head is held straight and eyes are level

- Chin is straight

- Shoulders are even

- Spaces (what I call "windows") between your arms and body are equal

- Thumbs are facing forward with palms facing the sides of your thighs
- Hips are level
- Kneecaps face straight ahead
- Feet are straight with a visible arch

YOUR ALIGNMENT IS OFF IF:

- The head tilts to one side or is pitched forward
- One shoulder is lower than the other, especially if it's your nondominant side
- Spaces between your arms and body are unequal
- Arms are in front, versus alongside of, the thighs
- Thumbs and palms are turned inward and facing backward when your arms are at your sides
- One hip is higher than the other
- Either or both of your kneecaps turn in or out
- Ankles and feet roll inward so weight is on the inner borders of the feet

KEEP YOUR HEAD UP AND YOUR BODY WILL FOLLOW

Standing tall adds an air of confidence to a woman, a visible aura that states, "I know where I'm going." Good posture can add inches to your height, prevent belly bulge and help you avoid a lifetime of aches and pains. Maintaining alignment also ensures a healthy and pain-free spinal column.

With perfect alignment you have a terrific advantage. You can move in any direction with a minimum of stress on your body. Your use of energy is efficient because you are holding yourself upright with muscles designed for that specific purpose. You look, and feel, great!

Being aligned means that your body follows the natural curves within it. A slight hollow in the lower back is maintained along with a gentle forward curve in the neck area and a backward curve in the upper back. The latter two curves are visible from a side view.

The natural spinal curves are located in the neck (cervical spine), the upper back (the thoracic spine) and the lower back (lumbar spine and sacrum). These curves, which form a gentle **S**-shape, function as your body's natural shock absorption system.[1

Your body should also have what I call a relaxed verticality. By this I mean that all the bones in the skeleton should be stacked in a certain way. If imaginary lines were dropped along your sides and front, from the top of your head to the soles of your feet, the lines would pass through certain anatomical landmarks.

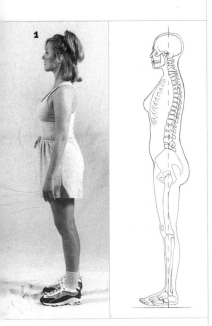

Ideal Posture

Viewing your body from each side, you would be able to see your ear aligned over your shoulder, the shoulder over the hip, and the hip in line with the side of your knee, the bony portion on the outside of your ankle. From the front, an imaginary line would run from right between your eyes, through your pelvis and between your knees and end up between the arches of your feet.

> *Christine, a 33-year-old makeup artist, stands much of the time during her typical workday. "I lean over people all day. At the end of the day my lower back is killing me; I can barely straighten up. The Core Program gave me much more stamina. I can stand for hours without thinking about it. My back pain is gone—and I stand tall at the end of the day."*
>
> *Christine stretched the muscles of the lower back and hips. She also stretched the vertebrae in her lower back, which relieved pressure and decompressed the vertebrae.*

THE CURVES THAT COUNT

In early fetal development, the spine is **C**-shaped. By the time a baby is one year old, three separate spinal curves develop. A forward curve, known as normal *cervical lordosis,* develops in the cervical spine. This curve is essential, as it keeps the head in position over the spine. Then, the thoracic spine, where the ribs are attached, forms a backward curve known as *kyphosis.* Finally, another forward curve called *lordosis* forms in the lumbar region in the lower spine. When these natural curves are altered because the body is out of alignment, four deviated postures occur that cause a multitude of problems. They are:

reversed neck lordosis, in which the head is thrust forward. This extreme position, which is common to all of the deviated postures, can change soft tissue and, over time, the bony contours of the spine, leading to the formation of a dowager's hump at the bottom of the neck as well as degeneration of the disks and facet joints as osteoarthritis progresses. Weakened neurological input to the arms is another result, as well as changes in jaw alignment that promote TMJ, teeth grinding and pain.

too much kyphosis, which is marked by the development of rounded shoulders and a caved-in appearance around the chest. This position can lead to a shortening of pectoral muscles as well as muscles lying between the ribs. This adaptive shortening weakens the overall stability of the shoulders, in addition to inhibiting effective breathing. [**2**

hyperlordosis, or swayback, which results when the normal forward curves of the cervical and lumbar spine are exaggerated, and the lower back arches excessively inward. This posture puts great

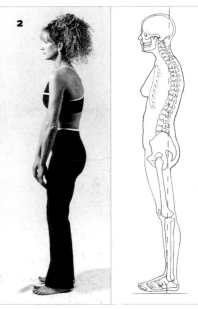

Kyphotic Posture

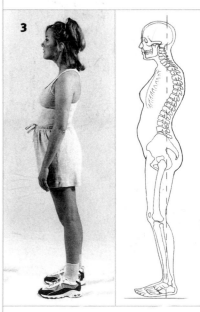

Swayback Posture

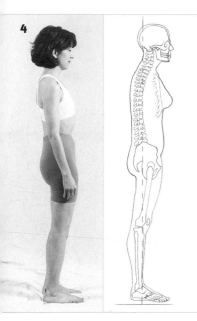

Flatback Posture

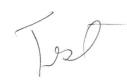

**Treating Another
Spine Curve**

Scoliosis, which is sometimes congenital, is a condition in which the spine curves to one side. My scoliosis patients respond to the Core Program, just as patients who favor one side—i.e., phone huggers—do.

strain on the lumbar vertebrae and on the adjacent joints between them. At the same time, the knees hyperextend, creating "bow" legs. The farther the belly hangs out, the greater the inward pull of the lower back, which increases the strain on the lower-back muscles and triggers painful muscle tightness and spasm. Also, excessive pressure is unequally distributed along the vertebral disks. Some disks begin to wear out prematurely, and lose their ability to absorb shock. Arthritis develops. Pregnancy exaggerates this posture, leading to back pain. [3

no lordosis, or flatback, which is brought about by a backward tilt of the pelvis and diminished stride length, which then removes the normal lumbar curve from the spine. The result is that no curves can be seen in the lower back and the head is thrust too far forward. This posture causes neck and back strain, too. [4

START YOUR REALIGNMENT RIGHT NOW

Here's something you can do right now to improve your posture. The more you do it, even for short periods, the better your posture will become.

These simple steps will help to keep your body aligned when you walk.

- Stand straight.
- Hold your chin up, with your head centered between your shoulders, and keep your eyes looking straight ahead.
- Relax your shoulders.
- Fill your lungs with air. This will lift your chest and further relax the shoulders as you exhale.
- Pull your abdomen in toward your back.
- Swing your arms naturally, keeping them close to your body, with hands loose and unclenched. This helps maintain balance.
- Extend your legs in a comfortable stride.
- Give your feet the attention they deserve. If you don't, you won't be able to walk or stand efficiently.

WHEN SHOES FIT RIGHT, YOU STAND RIGHT

Properly supported feet help you move with maximum efficiency and encourage healthy spinal alignment. When you wear the right shoes, they provide both the firm support and the pliable flexibility that different areas of your feet require, and they also have a positive effect on the rest of you because every part of your body is affected by the way your feet hit the ground.

Finding shoes that will support your feet properly isn't difficult. To make sure you know what to look for, here are the basic facts about shoe construction.

- The *toe box* is the part of the shoe that provides space for the toes. It should not cramp either the length, depth or the width of your foot. To assure the shoe is the proper length, check that there is at least one-half inch of space between the tip of the shoe and your longest toe. Press down on the tip of the shoe and use the width of your thumbnail as a measure.

- The *sole* consists of an insole and an outsole. The insole is the inner surface of the shoe on which the foot rests; the outsole is the bottom of the shoe, which contacts the ground and helps provide traction. The better cushioned and more resilient the sole, the greater the shoe's ability to absorb shock.

- The *counter* is the back part of the shoe, which curves around the heel of the foot. The counter should be firm, to support the foot and give the rear foot stability when the heel strikes the ground during walking.

- The *heel*, which extends from the counter, provides elevation for a stable heel strike. In order to avoid excessive strain on the fore-foot, which can deform the toes, choose a heel between one and one and a half inches high. Shoes with heels shorter than this recommended height strain the arches of your feet, which can lead to plantar fasciitis and heel spurs.

No matter what kind of shoe you're buying, remember to think of the foot as a triangle. The weight-bearing heel and the first and fifth toes form the three points of the triangle. Your weight should be evenly distributed among these three points.

Be sure the toe box provides enough room for the widest part of your foot: The more a shoe mimics the shape of your foot, the less wear and tear on your feet. As you stand, the tips of your longest toes should be at least one-half inch from the end of the shoe, the counter of the shoes should fit snugly, and there should be shock-absorbent soles on the bottoms of the shoes. Look for shoes that offer comfortable, supportive arches and make sure the heels are between one and one and a half inches high.

Because foot size changes with age, you should have your feet remeasured every two years so you can adjust your shoe size. Have them measured in the afternoon when they are at their largest. If one foot is bigger than the other, buy shoes to fit the larger one. And remember to try on shoes with the same sort of socks or hose you plan to wear with them.

THOSE HEELS AREN'T MADE FOR WALKING

An ill-fitting pair of shoes can lead to a host of foot problems. A tight fit will eventually cause everything from corns to pinched nerves and permanent, painful thickening of soft tissues as well as bony deformities.

High heels exacerbate already existing foot problems common to

Your Feet Tell a Lot About You

Look at your feet. If your toe-nails are in good condition and your skin isn't cracked, dry or flaky, the blood flow to the feet is unrestricted. Hair on your toes is always a sign of healthy circulation.

53

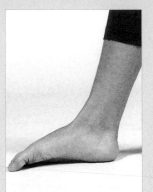

If you don't have strong arches, the fat pads under the toe knuckles can wear down and cause pain.

The Arch Builder. This exercise builds up the transverse arch, the area at the base of the knuckles of the feet, and helps prevent hammertoes.

- Stand in your bare feet.
- Take a half step forward with your right foot.
- With your right heel firmly on the floor and your toes as straight as possible, raise the top of your foot to create a dome. Hold for six seconds. Release.
- Switch to the other foot.
- Repeat three to six times.

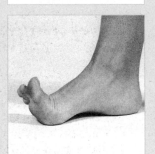

The Toe Lift. This exercise builds up the longitudinal arch which runs along the inside of the foot and helps prevent flat feet.

- Still standing, lift the toes of both feet up while keeping the rest of the foot flat on the floor.
- Walk on the heels and balls of your feet with your toes lifted for three minutes.
- Do this daily to strengthen the arches of the feet.

Get a Little More Arch Support

Dr. Scholl's sandals for women have wooden soles with raised arch supports under the toe knuckles. Walking around in these shoes for fifteen minutes twice a day can strengthen the foot muscles that assist in supporting your transverse arch. It will also help lessen toe deformities.

women. Constantly wearing these shoes can produce structural changes in the feet, worsen any existing abnormality and may bring about enough injury to eventually necessitate surgery. In fact, nearly 90 percent of all foot surgery patients are women.

Heels higher than two inches force your body into an unnatural position by thrusting the lower back forward and upper back backward to maintain balance as well as increasing pressure behind your kneecap. They also cause a shift in the body's weight, placing it on the ball of the foot. The higher the heel, the greater the shift and the damage, since the foot bones assume drastically unnatural positions. As the heel rises in height, the foot's long bones become almost perpendicular to the floor and parallel to the leg bones. The harmful effects of heel height multiply when a narrow, pointy toe box crowds your toes.

The malalignments caused by wearing high heels increase stress on the lower back and knees, too. A recent study found that when women walked in heels, the forces exerted on the insides of their knees were 23 percent greater than when they strode barefoot. Over time, that's enough force to damage delicate knee cartilage and cause osteoarthritis.

There is also nerve damage to consider, due to the pinching caused by compressed foot bones. Constantly wearing high heels can adaptively shorten tendons, especially the ropelike Achilles tendon at the back of the ankle. High heels can also tighten calf muscles, resulting in heel pain and tendinitis, and can increase the risk of injury from trips and falls.

So I strongly suggest that you give up the high heels for daily use and stick with pumps wide enough for maximum stability with a squared or rounded toe box and a heel no higher than an inch and a half. Limit high heel–wearing time and alternate them with good-quality sneakers or leather tie-ups with one-inch-thick heels for part of the day.

Still, I would never advocate throwing out your cherished high heels. Just keep them in reserve for those special occasions when you know that you'll be sitting—a lot.

Choose the Perfect Sneakers

You practically have to have a degree in engineering to understand all the ways athletic shoe manufacturers design the various components of foot support. To make things a lot easier when buying a pair of sneakers, here's what you need to do.

First, stand, with your socks on, on one foot. Note your balance. Then put a sneaker on the same foot and stand on it again. Your balance should be the same—or better—than it was barefoot. Next, hop in place five times. If the sneaker fits properly you should have good balance. If you don't, move on to another pair until you find a sneaker that is right for you.

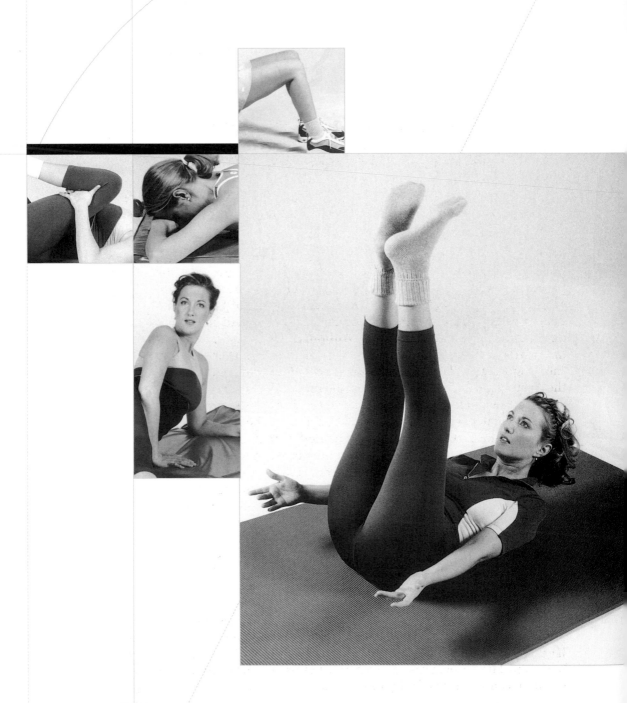

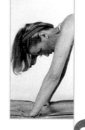

knowing your "hot spots"

chapter five

Many of my patients are referred to me by doctors. This often happens at the stage where the doctor has ruled out any serious pathology through various diagnostic tests such as MRIs, CAT scans, X-rays and blood tests, but is still unable to provide the patient with relief from the pain or discomfort that led her to the doctor's office in the first place. Although her symptoms might have mirrored those of a serious medical problem, there's really "nothing wrong" with her, or at least nothing that can be treated in the doctor's office. That's where I come in.

Once I evaluate the patient, I can usually trace the problem to muscle imbalances in the various "hot spots" of the body. To help you understand them better I've included a brief explanation of how the muscles and joints of each hot spot work together. Then, I've added a list of common injuries that occur at each hot spot, along with their symptoms. I view it as part of a core education.

Unless you actively work to correct them, muscle imbalances tend just to keep getting worse. Muscles that are too shortened resist being elongated, while overly elongated muscles contract with difficulty. When this happens, the joint that sits between these muscles is pulled out of its axis of rotation—which is what we mean when we say the joint is out of alignment.

Since we are adaptive beings, we create alternate movement patterns to compensate for these imbalances. Unfortunately, these patterns ultimately wear down not just the joints, but also the cartilage, the smooth, soft fibrous tissue that cushions bone against bone and allows pain-free movement. Premature deterioration of our joints and a vulnerability to injury are the result.

The hot spots are the:

- neck
- shoulder complex, including the upper back
- lower back
- abdominal zone
- pelvic area
- hips
- lower extremities, which include the knees, ankles and feet

  The Core Program offers lots of help for many different complaints stemming from "hot spot" imbalances. I've seen it relieve discomforts in:

  - *Helen, a 47-year-old who had difficulty climbing stairs*
  - *Margaret, a 39-year-old who suffered from groin pain*
  - *Joanna, who at 50 complained of a stiff back and was awakened at night by cramps in her calves*
  - *Donna, whose pregnancy at 35 gave her painfully swollen feet*
  - *Lynette, a 42-year-old whose feet felt cold all the time*

The Neck

Katie, a healthy, active 40-year-old, came to see me for the hand pain and weakness of carpal tunnel syndrome. "What I can't understand is that I worked on a typewriter for years and never had any hand problems," she told me. What Katie said gave me a big clue to the cause of her problem. Computer keyboards aren't spring-loaded like those on typewriters and the resulting vibration on the hands is different. The nerves in her hands were being compressed; also, she tended to lean her head forward as she worked, which took her neck out of alignment. The result was that the nerves in both her hands and her neck were being irritated. When I worked on her neck, she felt strength return to her hands right away. She did the Head-to-Toe Prep and the Butterfly from the Core Program and then progressed through the entire Core Foundation. After eight weeks she had 100 percent recovery.

You might think of your neck only as the column that supports your head. The neck does a lot more than that. Without neck movement you wouldn't be able to turn your head from side to side or lift it up to the night sky or tilt it down to read a book.

The neck contains seven vertebrae, stacked up like blocks, with blood vessels passing through the sides of each one. These blood vessels are responsible for the blood supply to your brain. To protect the vertebrae from rubbing against one another, there is a layer of cartilage between each bony surface. And to allow friction-free (and quiet) movement when you bend or rotate your neck, synovial fluid lubricates the interlocking joints. To further protect you, the disks between each vertebral segment act as shock absorbers.

The most mobile part of your spine, the neck depends on the integrity of your ligaments, as well as the strength of all your neck muscles, for balance. That balance is crucial because the position of the neck influences the movement and function of the head, jaw, upper back, shoulders and lower back.

So influential is the neck that every sensation and muscle contraction of your entire arm—down to the tips of your fingers—depends on nerves from your neck. This is why good alignment is so critical for optimal nerve and blood supply to all the muscles of your upper body.

The Head-to-Toe Prep in the Core Foundation and Intermediate Core, the Butterfly in all three programs, and the Mermaid in the Intermediate and Ultimate Cores are all good exercises to do to keep the nerves and muscles of your upper body working as they should.

When your neck isn't functioning optimally, here's what can happen:

SIGNS AND SYMPTOMS OF NECK DYSFUNCTION

Fatigue and/or weakness in arms and/or hands
Shoulder tension
Shoulder "popping"
Cold hands
Pins-and-needles feeling in hands

COMMON DIAGNOSES

Neck strain
Whiplash
Osteophytes (bony spurs)
Degenerative disk disease
Carpal tunnel syndrome
Shoulder strain
Tennis elbow
Headaches
Neck pain
Grinding teeth
Difficulty swallowing
Ringing in ears
Jaw pain
Twitching eyes

The Shoulder Complex and the Upper Back

Only 25, Tamar complained of tightness along her upper back near the right shoulder, which extended down into her right arm. "I ache right here," she showed me, vigorously rubbing her shoulder. "It hurts so much that it disturbs my concentration. I even have trouble finding a comfortable position when I sleep."

When I asked Tamar to raise her right arm straight up over her head she was amazed that she couldn't do it. Then she confessed that she had trouble clasping a bra behind her and that even using the hair dryer left her right shoulder feeling tired. She also reported arm weakness when reaching over to tune the car radio.

It turned out that Tamar hunched forward when she read, thereby tensing and straining her neck muscles. Also, since she was right-handed, she always carried her heavy leather briefcase on her right shoulder. Like most of us, she was overusing her "dominant" side.

By repeating these actions day after day, she was forcing the disks in her spine to abnormally press on nerves, compressing and entrapping them. I suggested that Tamar think of a kink in a garden hose. "When it gets tangled, water flows through slowly, in spurts, instead of in a steady stream," I explained. In Tamar's case, the electrical impulses that traveled within her shoulder weren't reaching the muscles and they, in turn, couldn't work effectively.

Also, because using her shoulder was so painful, she stopped moving it unless she really had to. Unfortunately, this made things worse; she had, in effect, "frozen" her shoulder joint.

In addition to physical therapy techniques, the exercises of the Core Program helped Tamar's shoulder heal and recover. By exercising the muscles for proper postural alignment, Tamar was able to move her shoulder without discomfort. Tension was relieved in "tight" areas and pressure was taken off the nerves in her lower neck. At the same time, strength returned to her right arm.

The shoulder girdle is a complex of four joints—the acromioclavicular, the scapulothoracic, the sternoclavicular and the glenohumeral—whose functioning is dependent on the strength and balance of the muscles surrounding them. There are three major muscle groups that connect to the shoulder joints: 1) the shoulderblade muscles, which consist of the levator scapulae, upper, middle and lower trapezius, the serratus anterior, the rhomboids, major and minor, and the latissimus dorsi; 2) the chest muscles, which are made up of the pectorals, major and minor; 3) the deltoids and the four muscles of the rotator cuff. The four muscles of the rotator cuff insert into the shoulder and hold it up. (You know how it feels when you put your arm around someone's shoulder and rest your hand on top of it? That's how the muscles of the rotator cuff cup the joint and hold your arm against the shoulder blade.)

The four joints of the shoulder complex allow for multidirectional movements, while the muscles around them act as stabilizers and generate all the power to the arms.

The *acromioclavicular* (AC) joint is the structure that connects the collarbone (clavicle) to the shoulder blade (scapula). It provides a protective roof for the rotator cuff, tendons and the bursa (the sac between tendons and bone that contains lubricating fluid).

The *scapulothoracic* joint, between the upper back and the shoulder blade, gives the shoulder girdle stability and ideal joint alignment. It attaches the shoulder blade to the back of the torso.

The *sternoclavicular* joint attaches the collarbone to the chest wall at the sternum. This joint helps keep arm motions smooth and nerves unobstructed while the collarbone moves back and forth and up and down.

The *glenohumeral* joint is a ball-and-socket–like structure that rotates to allow the shoulder to move in all directions. But if the muscles controlling the alignment of the other three joints that make up the shoulder girdle are not well balanced, the ball-and-socket becomes dysfunctional.

One of the exercises I recommend for strengthening the back muscles and aligning the shoulder joints is the Butterfly, which is included, with variations, in all three Core Programs.

When your shoulder isn't functioning optimally, here's what can happen:

SIGNS AND SYMPTOMS OF SHOULDER DYSFUNCTION

Trouble lifting overhead
Trouble reaching behind you (e.g., to fasten your bra)
Pain with any kind of carrying, pushing or pulling
(even pulling up panty hose)
Trouble sleeping on affected side
Popping and clicking shoulder noises
Upper-back pain

COMMON DIAGNOSES

Bursitis
Frozen shoulder
Tendinitis
Rotator cuff tear
Shoulder impingement
Dislocation (a joint totally out of alignment)
Subluxation (a joint partially out of alignment)
Bone spurs
Cartilage tears

The Lower Back

Debra, 39, first noticed the discomfort as she was getting out of a chair at a dinner party. "Initially, I didn't think about it. After all, the chair was big and deep," she told me on her first visit. "Now, however, I realize I'm having this pain a lot of the time. I have trouble sitting at my desk for even half an hour. Also, my legs feel tired all the time even though I'm not walking that much. What's the matter with me?"

Because of Debra's sedentary lifestyle, muscles in her lower back, hips and buttocks had shortened and badly needed to be stretched. With the Core Program she was able to improve flexibility, which made her legs feel better right away. At the same time her spine was stretched and elongated, allowing nerves to relay fully their messages to muscles in her lower extremities. This made it much easier for Debra to raise herself out of a chair. The core exercises realigned her spine and hips to allow proper movement to occur and relieve her pain.

By the time 36-year-old Melanie came to see me, she had been experiencing intermittent lower-back pain for a couple of years. Now pain was radiating down her right leg. "I had an MRI to rule out a herniated disk and nothing significant showed up," she told me.

When Melanie told me about her intense weekend gardening I determined that some of the positions she constantly assumed were exerting pressure on disks, ligaments and nerve roots in her back. This was the source of her pain. So she first had to use the exercises of the Core Program to undo these problems, and then, before going back to her former activities, she had to learn new ways of bending and kneeling and lifting and carrying.

With the Core Program, Melanie strengthened weak muscles and stretched to decompress the spaces between the disks in her lower back. As a result, the nerves were no longer being trapped against disks. Tension in her spine was relieved and normal function was restored. An additional benefit of the program was that she could stand straight without discomfort after all her kneeling. And her arms became stronger too, which allowed her to spend more time in her garden.

The backbone, also known as the spinal column, gives us the ability to stand, and sit, upright. Running the length of the back, from the base of the skull to the tip of the coccyx, the spinal column encases and protects the spinal cord. The spinal cord is the major nerve impulse highway that transmits messages to and from the brain, and then out to the muscles of the arms and legs. Together with the brain, the 1.5-ounce spinal cord forms the central nervous system.

Thirty-one pairs of major nerve roots emerge from each side of the spinal cord, dividing into the motor nerves, which enable the muscles to contract and expand, and the sensory nerves, which allow you to perceive sensations of touch, temperature and pain. The largest nerve group in the lower extremities is the sciatic nerve, which consists of five nerve roots that emerge from each side of the lumbar spine, then pass through the buttocks and down each leg all the way to the toes. Many different kinds of leg pain are referred to as "having sciatica," though that's really just a description of where the pain is felt, not a diagnosis of what caused it.

The spine is divided into three separate sections comprised of thirty-three cylindrical blocks of bone, or vertebrae. There are seven cervical vertebrae in the neck, twelve thoracic vertebrae in the upper and middle back (each has a pair of ribs attached) and five lumbar vertebrae in the lower back. These lumbar vertebrae are designed to support your back, as well as absorb the stresses of sitting, standing and walking. At the very bottom of the spinal column are the nine smaller vertebrae, which comprise the sacrum and the coccyx. The sacrum attaches the pelvis to the spine.

All spinal stability depends on two sets of forces: the passive constraints of ligaments, cartilage and all the bony connections; and the active constraints of muscles. We can improve our spinal stability by working the muscles of the lower back, through such exercises as the Butterfly and the Cross Extension, both of which appear in the Core Foundation. We can also reduce tension and pressure on the lower-back muscles by stretching them, which is why I've included the all-important Cobra in each of the Core Programs.

When your lower back isn't functioning optimally, here's what can happen:

SIGNS AND SYMPTOMS OF LOWER-BACK DYSFUNCTION

Pain when reaching
Pain during or after sports
Quick, sharp pain
Trouble standing upright after bending or sitting
Weak legs
Difficulty walking
Trouble lifting

Limited movement
Radiating leg pain

COMMON DIAGNOSES

Sciatica
Strains (muscles)
Sprains (ligaments)
Spasms
Disk herniations, bulges or ruptures
Spinal stenosis (narrowing of nerve passageways)
Osteoporosis
Osteoarthritis
Osteophytes (bone spurs)
Degenerative disk disease
Degenerative joint disease

The Abdominal Zone

Vivian loves doing ballroom dancing; being active is an important part of this 57-year-old's lifestyle. She was increasingly bothered, however, by painful "stitches" in her side whenever she danced. "It's the oddest thing," she told me. "My doctor checked me out and said I was fine. I feel okay—but if I'm okay, why should I be having pain?" I traced Vivian's discomfort to a weakened abdominal zone. Once she started strengthening the all-important muscles there, those annoying "stitches" were gone.

The four abdominal muscles are the rectus abdominis, the obliques, both internal and external, and the transverse abdominis.

RECTUS ABDOMINIS

This long, flat muscle extends along the entire length of the front of the torso from the pubic bone up to the rib cage with horizontal tendons fanning out to the right and left. When people refer to "six-pack abs" they are talking about a buffed rectus abdominis.

The rectus abdominis inserts into the sternum and attaches to the fifth, sixth and seventh ribs. The linea alba, a tendonlike structure, separates the right and left halves of this muscle. During pregnancy, the linea alba separates to make abdominal room for the growing baby and expanding uterus. This separation of the rectus abdominis, which is called a diastasis recti, is expected to close completely six to twelve months after the baby is delivered.

When you want to lie down or get up, sit down or sit up, the rectus abdominis helps you do so by flexing your trunk and drawing your breastbone toward your pubic bone.

THE OBLIQUE MUSCLES

The *external obliques* are the largest and most superficial of your abdominals. They run along the front and both sides of the

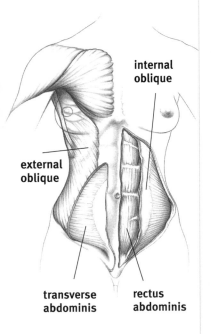

internal
oblique

external
oblique

transverse
abdominis

rectus
abdominis

abdomen from the lower eight ribs, and insert into the crest of your pelvis. These muscles help flex, bend and rotate your spine.

The muscles come inward and meet the horizontal tendons of the rectus abdominis almost like a pair of hands, with fingers flared, holding in your flanks. When you strengthen these muscles your waistline gets smaller.

The *internal oblique* muscles, located just under the external obliques, mimic the function of their partners.

TRANSVERSE ABDOMINIS

Called the "girdle" muscle, the transverse abdominis, a deep muscle under the obliques, attached to the spine, supports the lower abdomen and pelvic organs and stabilizes the spine. For several reasons, it is very important to strengthen this muscle. Doing so will prevent both lower-back pain and urinary incontinence. It will also help ease bowel movements, because the transverse abdominis muscle can create pressure on the intestines—think of toothpaste being squeezed from the tube. Pregnant women greatly

Stop Forcing Yourself to Do Sit-ups, Curl-ups and Crunches

Performing any or all of this trio will strengthen your abdominal muscles—but at too high a cost. These exercises push your head forward out of alignment, trigger tension in the upper shoulder and actually weaken the transverse abdominis, causing it to pouch. That's why these movements won't flatten your belly. The other major problem with these exercises is that they can lead to urinary stress incontinence due to excessive pressure on the pelvic floor.

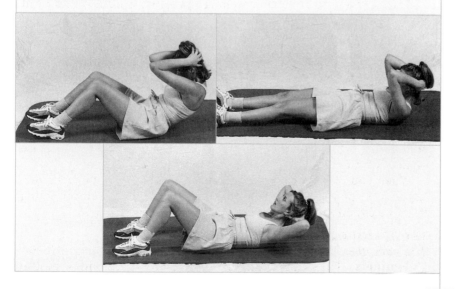

benefit from a toned transverse abdominis because the muscle supports the weight of the baby in the pelvis. The muscle also assists in pushing the baby out during delivery. And if all of these benefits aren't enough, a strong transverse abdominis means a flatter belly!

While all the movements in the Core Program exercise the abdominals, the Belly Blaster in the Core Foundation, and Dead Bugs and the Mermaid in the Intermediate Core and Double Dead Bugs and the Advanced Mermaid in the Ultimate Core, specifically train abdominals to work the way you need them to work. That means being able to recruit your abs when you reach, lift and carry—all the things you do in the course of a day.

When your abdominal muscles aren't functioning optimally, here's what can happen:

SIGNS AND SYMPTOMS OF ABDOMINAL DYSFUNCTION

Lower-back pain
"Stitches" in side when active
Poor bladder control

COMMON DIAGNOSES

Hernia
Diastasis recti
Urinary stress incontinence
Recurring back strains
Unrelenting lower-limb spasms

The Pelvic Floor

Forty-one-year-old Lea came to my office complaining about lower-back pain that tended to come and go. But once we started to talk, she expressed a greater concern: her loss of bladder control. "I can't believe this is happening," she told me. "I thought only elderly women had this problem. My gynecologist checked me out thoroughly and determined that there's nothing physically wrong with me. That's what doesn't make sense. Why should I have 'accidents' if everything is okay?"

It turned out that the cause of Lea's urinary incontinence stemmed from repetition of a very popular exercise. After ten years of faithfully performing abdominal "crunches," she had unintentionally weakened the muscles of her pelvic floor. As a result, she was experiencing mild urinary stress incontinence whenever she coughed, sneezed or even laughed.

I advised Lea to stop doing crunches and substitute Dead Bugs, one of the core exercises, instead. By doing so

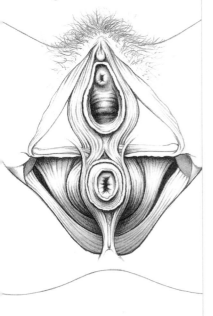

The muscles of a woman's pelvic floor, surrounding and supporting the urethra, the vagina and the rectum.

Lea was able to build maximum abdominal strength without putting strain on the pelvic floor. Her urinary stress incontinence disappeared—and she is secure in the knowledge that it won't return.

The pelvic floor is the band of three muscles and connective tissue around the vagina and the anus. It controls both the anal sphincter and the urethral sphincter—the latter being the muscle that both stops the flow of urine and contracts during orgasm. The pelvic floor supports all the organs between the pubic bone and tailbone, not unlike a grocery bag. And like the bottom of that grocery bag, the bottom of the supporting structure of the pelvic floor needs to be strong.

Kegels for Pelvic Strengthening

The Core Program will give you the pelvic toning you need. However, if you want to do some additional pelvic strengthening, there are exercises known as Kegels, which focus exclusively on the urethral sphincter, also known as the pubococcygeal muscle. If you would like to start Kegels, follow the instructions below regarding the two basic variations. Perform them for one to two weeks in each of the following positions before progressing to the next position.

To begin, perform these exercises lying on your back. (You can add a pillow under your buttocks if you wish.)

Then advance to lying on your back with your knees bent and your pelvis tilted up.

Next, perform the exercises while sitting (the possibilities are endless: at the theater, while driving, at meetings—no one will ever know!).

After doing sitting Kegels, progress to a standing position (for once, waiting in line can be put to practical use).

Finally, do the exercises in squatting positions on the floor or over the toilet.

1. Closing and Opening Flower

Tighten your sphincter muscles, which surround the urethra, vagina and rectum, like a flower closing its petals.

This is the same feeling you have when you need to urinate but must "hold" it in. Do not tighten your buttocks or abdominal muscles. Hold for six seconds and release, or "open," slowly. Repeat six times.

2. Elevator Going Up

Tighten your sphincter muscles and then lift up between the vagina and rectum. Lift to the top floor and hold for three seconds. Release slowly, one floor at a time. Do this contract-and-go-up exercise once, six times a day.

There is another Kegel exercise that requires a partner. Sexercise, as its name suggests, is performed during intercourse. With your legs spread and relaxed, grip the penis as firmly as possible with your vagina. Hold for three to six seconds before relaxing. Remember to avoid tensing your buttocks and/or abdominal muscles—and do ask your partner for feedback.

To test that you're doing it right, before intercourse insert two fingers in the entrance of the vagina and squeeze. If you feel pressure you are doing this muscle contraction correctly.

Strengthening the pelvic floor will enhance sexual pleasure, and it will also help a problem that has reached near epidemic proportions—urinary stress incontinence. This is not a subject that gets a lot of attention, but it should, because it affects a surprising number of younger women as well as the elderly, and not just women who are weak or out of shape. It is known that women who exercise vigorously can leak anywhere from a few drops to a half cup of urine during a workout session. A recent study of 144 female varsity college athletes between the ages of 18 and 21 revealed that 28 percent experienced leakage at some point while performing their sport.

Another study of nearly 300 female recreational exercisers between the ages of 17 and 68 revealed that a third of them experienced incontinence during exercise. An additional 20 percent stopped exercising because of incontinence, while another 18 percent modified their workouts or exercise because of it. Incredibly, more than half the group wore protective pads while exercising.

What causes the prevalence of this condition? It's not always curls, crunches and sit-ups, of course. Childbirth, obesity and abdominal surgery—anything that contributes to the loss of strength in the pelvic floor and lower abdominal muscles—can all cause urinary incontinence. When these muscles are stretched and lose their power, the ability of the urinary sphincter to hold urine in the bladder is compromised.

Two core exercises are particularly beneficial to pelvic floor muscles: Dead Bugs in the Intermediate Core, and Double Dead Bugs in the Ultimate Core.

When your pelvic floor isn't functioning optimally, here's what can happen:

SIGNS AND SYMPTOMS OF PELVIC FLOOR DYSFUNCTION

Urinary stress incontinence—urine leaks when coughing, sneezing and/or laughing, running or jumping

Inability to reach orgasm, or weak orgasm

Painful sex

The Hips

When I first met Valerie I found it hard to reconcile the slim 32-year-old with the color photograph she showed me. Two years prior to her visit, Valerie had carried 225 pounds on her five foot, six inch frame. Working twice a week with a nutritionist and three times a week with a trainer, she had lost nearly one hundred pounds and many inches.

"I have a strange complaint," she began, "and I don't know what to do about it. When I was heavy, I walked a certain way. To be perfectly honest, I waddled. Instead of lifting my legs, I sort of slid my feet out to the side, one after the other. Now that I'm thin—and fit—I still do it. Sometimes I even catch myself limping. Why am I doing this?"

Valerie's complaint is more prevalent than she ever imagined. Many women without weight problems who sit throughout the day trigger an imbalance of the muscles around their hips. Walking becomes difficult; many couldn't run even if they wanted to. Others feel a pinch in the groin.

I did a manual muscle test on Valerie and found a consistent weakness in her gluteus medius, the pelvis-hip muscle. This kind of weakness can create a limp or waddle. I told Valerie that stabilizing her spine and hip muscles was necessary to allow her gluteus medius to work at full capacity.

Using the Core Program, Valerie stabilized her spine and stretched her hips while simultaneously bolstering the muscles in her torso. The result was that Valerie's waddling gait disappeared.

Think of your hips as your body's shock absorbers and you'll get an accurate idea of the significant role they play. The hips are the strongest joints in your body; they support all your weight when you are upright. The hips, along with the pelvis, allow for power and a full stride when you walk. The rotational ability provided by the hips allows you to move your torso through a wide range of motion. Otherwise, it would be left to your ankles, knees and spine to absorb the shock waves that rumble through you with every step. Just as important, hips also absorb some of the stresses that come from standing upright, walking and sitting throughout the day.

The hip is the point at which the thighbone meets the three bones that make up each side of the pelvis: the sit bones, hipbone and pubic bone. Like the glenohumeral shoulder joint, the hips are ball-and-socket joints, but they are much deeper and more stable.

Heel Beats and the Three-Part Pelvic Stabilizer, both of which appear in all the Core Programs, are particularly effective at strengthening hip muscles.

When your hips aren't functioning optimally, here's what can happen:

SIGNS AND SYMPTOMS OF HIP DYSFUNCTION

Leg weakness
Buttock pain
Trouble climbing stairs
Back pain
Groin pain
Overly short stride

Trouble running
Difficulty walking
Trouble lying on involved side

COMMON DIAGNOSES

Bursitis
Tendinitis
Impingement
Osteoarthritis
Osteoporosis

The Lower Extremities

The Knees, Ankles and Feet

"I love going to the theater, ballet, opera, concerts—you name it, I'm there," 48-year-old Becky told me. "Only now, my attention is distracted. It's my knees—I can't sit for long periods of time in those cramped seats without feeling pain."

I found that Becky's knee joints were considerably out of alignment. With the Core Program, Becky was able to strengthen and balance her upper-leg muscles as well as her abdominals, which helped realign her knees and also enabled her to reap all the other rewards of doing the exercises. Her knees are so improved she can now easily walk two miles every day.

At 53, Fern accompanied every movement into and out of her car with the same defeated sigh of discomfort. When the whiplash of a fender bender brought her to my office, she told me that her right knee always ached. "I know it's a sign of aging," she stated flatly. "I've had to give up bowling, which I really enjoy. I've played with the same team for years."

I asked if her left knee hurt her, too.

"No," she answered. "Should it?"

"No," I informed her, "it shouldn't. Our bodies age symmetrically. You can't have an 'old' right knee and a 'young' left knee. There's no reason why your right knee—and its companion—can't function painlessly for your entire life." The strengthening exercises of the Core Program resolved Fern's right-knee pain while ensuring that the left one would not weaken. Once again she bowls with her buddies every week.

The knee is a hinge joint, which connects the two rounded surfaces of the large thighbone (femur) with the lower shinbone (tibia). With only slight rotational movement, the knee joint moves backward and forward, making it possible for you to turn on a dime, and then to run off again at full speed without giving the matter a second thought. Because of its role as the link between femur and tibia, the knee is in particular need of both stability and mobility, which it gets from ligaments and from the quadriceps, the large muscles in the front of the thighs. Several powerful ligaments—think of them as sturdy ropes—hold the knee together. The two collateral ligaments hold the knee on the inside and outside, while the anterior and posterior cruciate ligaments crisscross inside the joint.

The four quadriceps muscles assure proper kneecap alignment by pulling equally on the kneecap, which, in turn, then acts as an efficient lever, giving greater power and control to the quadriceps. The quadriceps also help absorb all the ground-force shocks to the upper body.

The thin layer of articular cartilage covers the bones while the menisci protect and cushion the knee from wear and tear. The menisci absorb shock to the knees especially when you go up and down stairs, jump or twist. These gristlelike substances lie between the femur and tibia and keep the bones from rubbing against each other. Proper muscle balance around the knee joint protects the menisci and cartilage from damage.

Farther down from the knee sits the vulnerable ankle joint. The ankle bone, called the talus, along with the ends of the two lower-leg bones, forms the ankle joint. Two groups of ligaments, one on each side of the ankle, stabilize it.

And finally, there are your feet, each with twenty-six bones, nineteen muscles and 107 ligaments.

Steel Thighs, which is part of the Four-Part Progressive Hamstring Stretch in both the Core Foundation and the Intermediate Core, helps strengthen the quadriceps. In the Ultimate Core, squats are particularly beneficial to the entire lower extremities, especially the quadriceps.

When your lower extremities aren't functioning optimally, here's what can happen:

SIGNS AND SYMPTOMS OF KNEE DYSFUNCTION

Swelling in knees or ankles
Difficulty walking
Trouble putting weight on leg
Pain sitting still for short period
Inability to jump
Weakness in legs
Pain going up steps
Trouble kneeling
Grinding kneecap
Clunking sounds
Feeling of instability

COMMON DIAGNOSES

Cartilage tears
Ligament sprains
ACL tear
Chondromalacia
Patellofemoral dysfunction
Hamstring pull
Osteoarthritis
Tendinitis

SIGNS AND SYMPTOMS OF ANKLE DYSFUNCTION

Swelling
Pain
Weakness

COMMON DIAGNOSES

Achilles rupture
Sprains
Strains
Tendinitis
Heel spurs
Runner's Bump Pump

SIGNS AND SYMPTOMS OF FOOT DYSFUNCTION

Heel pain
Pain along toes
Pain while walking
Pain while standing
Abnormal gait
Burning sensation
Pins and needles

COMMON DIAGNOSES

Bunions
Calluses
Hammertoes
Morton's neuroma
Plantar fascitis

Now that you know something about your body's hot spots, and how they can lead to trouble, it's time to do something about them. If you need further encouragement to embark on the Core Program, read the following chapter, which will reassure you about the fact that these exercises will work for *all* women, of all ages, sizes, shapes and degrees of fitness. If you're raring to go, then proceed directly to the Core Foundation and get started on building the strong core you need.

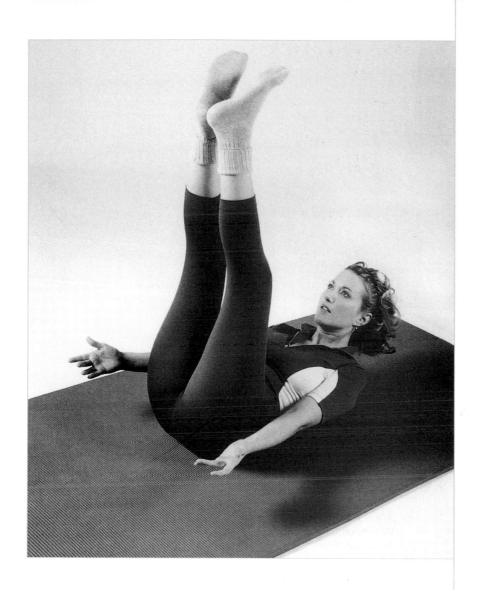

focus on change

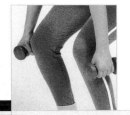

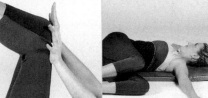

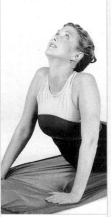

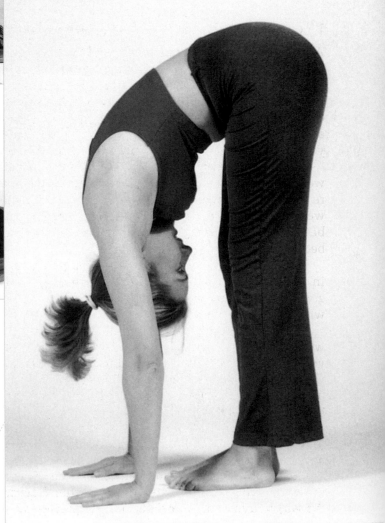

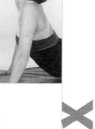

prepare your mind and your body will follow

chapter six

THE CORE PROGRAM: IT'S RIGHT FOR YOU

Among the many wonderful aspects of the Core Program is the one that is perhaps the most important of all: It is for every woman. If you haven't exercised in years, hate the idea of going to a gym and imagine that you can't do the movements, let me reassure you. The Core Program can be done anywhere. If you are more comfortable at home, that's the right place for you to exercise. Once you begin you will be amazed at what you can do in a very short time.

If you are carrying around extra pounds and believe that your weight is contributing to any aches and pains you may have, let me reassure you. I have treated women who were significantly over-weight and they have responded to the Core Program. They did so because their musculoskeletal imbalances were alleviated—not because they lost weight.

If you think you are too old, let me reassure you. I have patients in their eighties who do the Core Program and wouldn't dream of giving it up. Increased mobility, better posture, greater strength—why would they give that up?

If you exercise regularly, and include aerobic workouts and/or weight training in your regimen, I applaud your efforts and urge you to keep up the great work. But let me reassure you, too: The Core Program is the ideal complement to any exercise program because it protects the body against injury. If you wish, you can do the Core Program at the gym.

And if you don't do any exercise other than the Core Program, let me reassure you: Performing the movements will give your body the core benefits it needs.

If all this isn't enough motivation for you, consider this: Doing the Core Program will alter the way you function, as well as the way you feel, in your daily life. By preserving your joints and optimally strengthening your muscles, you will restore your body so that it works the way you need, and want it, to work.

I know that starting something new—much less finding the time for it—can take some doing. You're in overdrive the moment the clock radio turns on. There's a job to get to, children to prepare for school, carpooling, business presentations and entertaining. You're trying hard to remember your kids' play dates and whether you've stocked the fridge with everyone's favorites. Just trying to catch your breath by the end of the day can seem overwhelming.

That's why the Core Program is for you. All it requires is fifteen minutes a day, five times a week. And the returns on that quarter hour are tremendous. You will have all the energy you need to get through your day. You'll sit or stand, walk or lift, without any discomfort. You won't be bothered by aches and pains. You will be able to do everything you must do without a thought about where your strength is coming from. When your hectic day is done you will get a good night's sleep and awake recharged, ready to face the new day.

> *"I'm always on the go, with a full-time job, a husband and two children under ten, so making time for myself is never easy," 37-year-old Catherine told me. "However, I've found that doing the Core Program has energized me, as well as relieved those occasional aches and pains. If I'm running late and can't do my exercises after I get out of bed, I know I will do them sometime during the day. I've closed my door and done them in my office and I've also used the company gym. I know that taking those fifteen minutes for myself isn't selfish because so many people benefit from my being alert and strong. But I will say this: My body has changed in ways I never expected. I've lost inches and gained definition in my upper legs and arms. I've even been able to tone a place I'd given up on: Now I actually have that sexy indentation along the sides of my buttocks. Why would I ever stop doing the Core Program?"*

THE CORE PROGRAM AT A GLANCE

The first part of the program, the Core Foundation, should be done for at least three weeks before proceeding to the next part. But it won't take that long for you to notice a difference. In just one week you will feel better, stand taller and get a boost in strength. Just two weeks after that you will see changes brought on by using your body weight as resistance against gravity. Then, you will be feeling so much stronger and more confident in what your body can do that I bet you will be eager to try the Intermediate Core.

The Intermediate Core Program builds on what you've learned. With greater power and flexibility, you will be able to execute more difficult versions of some exercises, repeat others with improved range of motion and perform new ones with little or no problem. The Intermediate Core should also be performed for a minimum of three weeks. In this segment, you'll be using one- to two-pound ankle weights in a few of the exercises. These help to give your legs more definition as they help to diminish "saddlebags." Your body will become stronger and more toned as muscle replaces fat, and your body will become even more aligned. After three weeks, you may feel ready for the Ultimate Core.

The Ultimate Core is the most advanced level of the Core Program—and the goal to work toward. In this segment, you'll use two- to five-pound ankle weights, and in several exercises you'll also be using two- to five-pound dumbbells. You will receive a super toning effect along with an amazing boost in strength and stamina. Using weights can also make it easier to shed pounds and inches because weight training revs up your metabolic rate, thereby letting you burn more calories no matter what you are doing—even sitting or sleeping. At the same time, more lean muscle tissue and less fat result in a trimmer body, because fat takes up more room than the equal weight of muscle.

Soon after you begin, your body will become familiar with the movements and within just a few weeks they will become as routine as brushing your hair. You will find that you have created a new habit, one that will make you feel good every time you do it. When that happens, you will look forward to your "core" time. And as you continue to do the exercises, your appearance will change and your confidence will soar.

> "Before starting the Core Program I always had a weak back," 40-year-old Janice reported to me. "Even though I exercised regularly at the gym I always felt a backache coming on when I had to stand for longer than ten minutes. I realized that something was missing in my workouts— and the Core Program provided what I needed."
>
> Janice was so right. The Core Program strengthened her back muscles while helping to nourish the muscles by increasing blood flow. At the same time she was "stretching" the spaces between the lower vertebrae and relieving compression on nerves.

ALL YOU NEED TO GET STARTED

An exercise mat and comfortable clothes (no shoes!) that allow easy movement are all that is required to begin the Core Program. When you progress to the Intermediate and Ultimate Cores, it's time to invest in dumbbells and ankle weights.

Dumbbells. Choose among vinyl covered models, antiroll hexagonal head, or a set of shiny chrome-plated free weights. Please don't use substitutes, like soup cans, for dumbbells. Any can

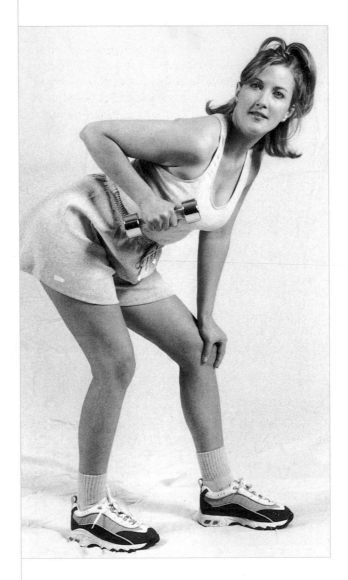

weighing more than one pound will be too big, and unwieldy, to hold. When you use dumbbells you can be assured that the weights are consistent.

Ankle Weights. There are two types of ankle weights. One consists of a canvas strap-on device outfitted with individual compartments for bars of iron weights. Weight is adjusted by adding or subtracting the bars to the ankle cuff. The other type comes in nonadjustable weights of three or five pounds.

MAKE THE CORE PROGRAM A PART OF YOUR LIFE

Once you decide to start the Core Program, there are three easy ways to help you stay with it.

MAKE IT A TOP PRIORITY

Take a look at your calendar. If you're like me, you probably pay special attention to the priorities penciled in red. So, add the Core Program and give it a big circle. Once you begin the Core Program, it means you're committed to taking care of yourself. Those fifteen minutes will give you personal rejuvenation time, recharging you physically and mentally. You deserve those fifteen minutes. They represent caring for yourself, being loving to yourself and respecting your body.

CHOOSE A SPECIFIC WORKOUT TIME

To help make the Core Program a habit, designate a fairly specific time slot. Some of my patients prefer to exercise a few hours before going to sleep to unwind after a stressful day. Others, myself included, do the exercises in the morning when uninterrupted time is easier to find. The choice is yours. Still, a good way to help you to stick to your new regimen is to always exercise in the same place.

However, don't do the Core Program too soon after eating, as you may feel bloated and sluggish. Also, I don't recommend doing it just before you go to bed, as exercise stimulates hormonal release that may keep you awake.

ENLIST SUPPORT IF YOU NEED IT

While many women prefer to make the commitment by themselves, others like the idea of exercising together. Or, even if they can't do the Core Program together, the idea that a friend across town is also doing it can be a motivator. Some women form a "core" group at work and do the exercises together at a certain time during the day. Others schedule a get-together with neighbors. Some women make it a family time routine, where children and spouses join in.

GIVE YOURSELF A GOAL

Achieving a short-term goal can bolster your spirits and encourage you. I have seen these goals—and many others—accomplished in just a few weeks.

- walking two miles without stopping
- toning upper arms
- lifting children older than two years
- getting definition in your legs
- walking up—or down—stairs without knee pain
- losing an inch from your waistline
- playing soccer with the kids
- dancing at a twenty-fifth reunion
- playing eighteen holes of golf
- getting up in the morning without stiffness

What would make *you* feel—and function—better?

When You Should Stop Exercising

Use common sense when you exercise. If you feel ill, stop what you are doing. And remember: Any pain, weakness, numbness or pins-and-needles sensation that persists longer than two weeks should be checked out by your physician.

Bonnie, a competitive runner, was highly motivated when she came to see me as she was preparing for a marathon. "I've been training for several years," the 28-year-old informed me, "and I'm looking for something that will give me an edge and allow me more power to run faster and longer."

Doing the Core Program gave Bonnie a leg up on the competition. She strengthened her outer- and inner-thigh muscles, which kept her kneecaps in line, built up the muscles of her hips, worked her hamstring muscles, bolstered all of her gluteal (buttock) muscles and stabilized her spine in the process. "I feel like I've got a secret weapon," she told me after she won the race.

TRAIN YOUR MUSCLES: DON'T STRAIN YOUR JOINTS

When you start the Core Program you may feel mild muscle achiness as you do the exercises. That feeling should be gone when the fifteen-minute session is over.

Because the Core Program protects joints from injury and helps to alleviate existing injuries, you should not feel any joint pain during, or after, a workout.

YOU CAN STAY MOTIVATED

Even if you're committed to doing the exercises, and have all the best intentions of continuing with them, you may eventually reach a point where you begin to experience the "toos." These are the excuses you invent to appease your conscience when a workout is skipped: There's too much work to do, too much homework to go over with the kids and you feel too tired. Once in a while, of course, there is an unavoidable reason for not performing your regimen.

Still, to keep your "toos" from occurring too often, here are a few suggestions:

■ Remember that the Core Program is supposed to relieve stress, not cause it. Don't be too hard on yourself; missing a planned workout doesn't mean that you have lost all you gained. You haven't. Just get back to your regular routine as soon as possible.

■ Turn on the television. Even if you're not paying attention to what is on the screen, sometimes it helps to have background noise.

■ If you do the Core Program to music, try varying the selection.

■ Do the self-tests on pages 27–31 again and be amazed by the progress you've made.

IT'S TIME TO CHANGE YOUR LIFE

When you turn the page you will find the exercise regimen that will help you feel and look great—and keep you that way—for the rest of your life!

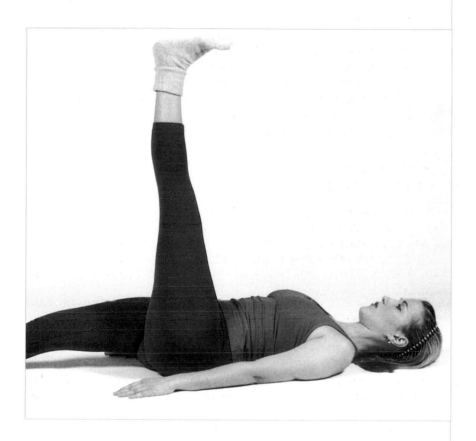

peggy brill's core program

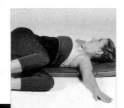

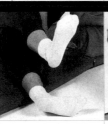

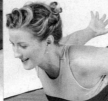

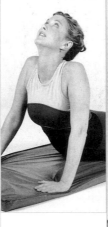

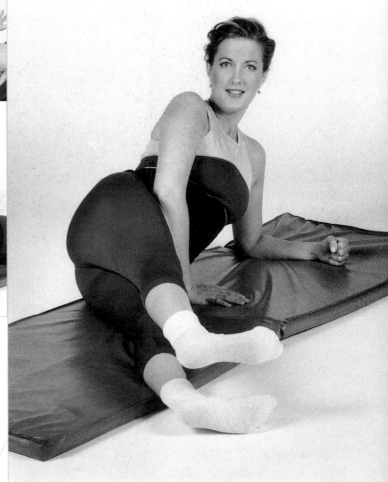

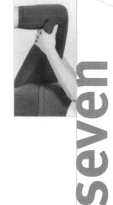

The Core Foundation

Here are the exercises that will change the way you feel and move and look for the rest of your life. They will do this because they were developed to first restore alignment, then enhance muscle flexibility and, ultimately, strengthen your body. Doing these exercises will also tone your body, giving your muscles new definition. Not only will you feel great as your posture straightens and you get stronger, you'll look great, too.

The exercises are targeted to all the various "hot spots" we've been discussing, as well as the abdominal zone, but doing them will alternately stretch and strengthen muscles throughout the entire body.

This alternation between pressure-off and pressure-on movements feels good, but even more important, it's good for you. Alternately tightening and releasing muscles will decrease the tension on the nerves within the muscle. When the nerve canals open, the nerves can deliver their electrical signals to the muscles more freely and muscles that had been foreshortened will become both longer and stronger. Simply stated, clenching a muscle ends up relaxing it. Here's an example: Many women feel tension in their shoulders at the end of the day. While the instinct is to stretch, the approach I use is different. Shrugging your shoulders and holding the position tightly for at least six seconds, then slowly relaxing, will ease the discomfort.

In addition to the obvious benefits that you get from being stronger, strong muscles help to keep your joints aligned, and well-aligned joints resist injury. A balanced joint is also likely to be well lubricated and therefore able to move freely. When joints are in alignment, there is no compression cutting off the flow of synovial fluid, the joints' lubricant.

The order in which the exercises appear, and the number of repetitions of each movement, are based on results I have seen in thousands of my patients. For example, I've mentioned the Head-to-Toe Prep several times in earlier chapters. The Core Foundation begins with this exercise because it is the perfect starting point for developing core stability. In a few brief movements the Head-to-Toe Prep elongates short muscles and strengthens muscles that are too long, thus creating balance. In essence, it sums up everything the Core Program does.

I've made sure the program requires the minimal number of reps necessary for achieving maximum results. Effective and efficient, the repetitions stretch and strengthen weakened muscles so that they work as they should and achieve balance with muscles that are already strong.

The Core Foundation is built mostly around isometric movements (also called static muscle contractions), which contract muscles without moving the joints attached to them. The strongest contractions a muscle can make, isometrics are the safest way to exercise because they avoid any joint irritation while they maximize recruitment of muscle fibers. Isometric strengthening of your core muscle groups assures spine stability.

Isotonic movements, which are used in exercising the extremities, involve movement of both the muscles and the joints. For instance, lifting weights is an isotonic form of exercise. Unfortunately, it's easy to injure yourself in a weight-lifting program because a weak muscle cannot keep a joint stable enough as it moves.

Because the Core Program focuses on isometric movements, it will not hurt your joints. You should know, however, that during the exercises tight muscles may feel a mild ache while they are being stretched. The discomfort should disappear when the exercise is over. If you feel pain that persists for two weeks, you should seek the advice of a medical professional.

A Core Concept

Recruiting Your Abdominal Muscles for Spinal Stability

Recruiting the abdominal muscles in the most effective way is key to getting the most out of the Core Program. As you lie flat on your back, follow these three steps for super abdominal recruitment:

1. Tilt your pubic bone up toward your navel while pulling your navel in to your spine. This movement recruits the lower abdominal muscles.
2. Pull your rib cage down toward your navel; you'll feel your back flattening against the mat. This movement recruits the upper abdominals. Your shoulders and head should stay relaxed on the mat.
3. Repeat the first movement. This targets the transverse abdominals and makes your efforts more effective. You'll be working not

only your abdominal muscles, but the muscles of your pelvic floor as well.

MAKE THE MOST OF YOUR WORKOUT

To maximize the effectiveness of your workout time, follow these guidelines:

EXERCISE SLOWLY AND STEADILY
Slow, controlled movements strengthen muscles most effectively. Quick, explosive movements may injure you.

USE A FULL RANGE OF MOTION
Be sure to move your body through the full range of motion the exercises indicate. Tightening muscles as much as possible will ultimately relax them and bring relief from spasms and cramping. Muscles that do only partial movement can lose flexibility.

HOLD FOR A MINIMUM COUNT OF SIX
Most of the exercises direct you to hold a position—that is, tighten your muscles—and then exhale for a count of six before releasing the position. I recommend that you count out loud. This will ensure that you are holding for the full count, and also that you are exhaling on exertion.

The reason for the six-second minimum hold has to do with the period of time it takes for nerve signals to travel to the brain. Tightening the muscle for six seconds or more maximizes the effect of relaxation in that muscle when you release it.

BE AWARE OF YOUR BREATHING AND
DON'T HOLD YOUR BREATH
Although most people aren't aware of holding their breath during an exercise, it's a very common response to exertion. The problem is that if you stop breathing while performing an exercise, you can give yourself muscle cramps and prevent blood from returning to your heart. You'll also make the work harder. So bring your attention back to your breath as you start each exercise, and keep breathing, always exhaling on exertion. Remember: Inhale and exhale through your nose—this helps filter the air. When you breathe through your mouth this doesn't happen.

TAKE A BELLY BREATH AND FEEL BETTER FAST

In addition to the normal breathing you should be sure to do during the exercises, I've included belly breathing breaks in all the Core Programs.

When you belly breathe, deep inhalations force your diaphragm, the muscle just beneath the lungs, to drop down. This action pushes your belly outward, creating a partial vacuum in the chest

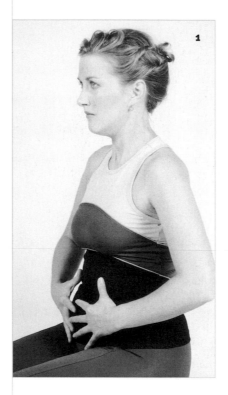

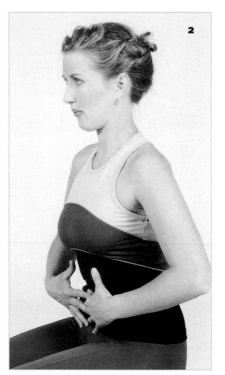

that will fill quickly with air. When you exhale, your diaphragm relaxes and the air is released. Belly breathing expands the muscles in the lower back, relieving muscle tension.

Just three or four deep belly breaths will signal your nerves to alert your heart, lungs, stomach and bladder muscles to relax. In addition to being an instant stress reducer, belly breathing can ease headaches, diminish fatigue, center emotions and help your mind to focus on a single activity.

You don't, however, have to wait to do the Core Program to take belly breaths. The cumulative effect of taking a few belly breaths every hour will make a huge difference in how you feel at the end of the day. Here's how it's done.

- Sit down, or lie on your back. Hold the palm of your hand against your stomach between your navel and rib cage. Breathe in deeply, 1–2–3–4. When you use your diaphragm to breathe, your stomach will push out against your hands. Hold this inhalation for seven seconds. [1

- Exhale slowly as you count to eight. You can feel your hand moving down as your stomach deflates. [2

- Practice this throughout the day, taking two to four deep breaths, through your nose, every hour. As you slowly exhale with the aid of your diaphragm, you'll feel your body unwind and muscular tension begin to flow out.

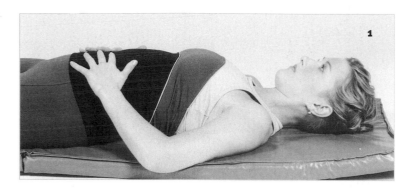

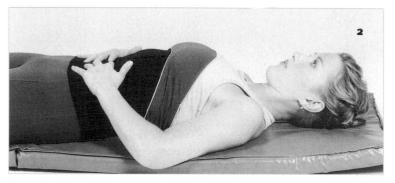

BEFORE YOU BEGIN

There is one thing you should always keep in mind: Unless otherwise stated, the exercises that are done while lying on your back are performed with your chin retracted, your abdominal muscles hollowed out and your pelvis slightly tilted.

I suggest that you look at both the directions and the photos to get a good understanding of how the different parts of an exercise flow together into a continuous sequence. Follow the instructions and pay attention to the "Form Checks" and "Tips." They offer reminders for quick adjustments to ensure that your form is right and that you are getting all the potential benefits of the program.

And a final reminder: Even if you passed all the self-tests on pages 27–31, you should still start with the Core Foundation. You should do it for one week, instead of the usual three, before progressing to the Intermediate Core. This way, you'll develop a greater awareness of the muscles that are supposed to do the work during these exercises.

1. Head-to-Toe Prep
2. Tongue Stretch
3. Belly Blaster
4. Belly Breath
5. The Cobra
6. Butterfly/Heel Beats Combo
7. Three-Part Pelvic Stabilizer
8. Four-Part Progressive Hamstring Stretch
9. Double Knees to Chest
10. Lying Spinal Twist
11. Belly Breath
12. Cross Extension
13. The Cobra
14. Belly Breath Finale

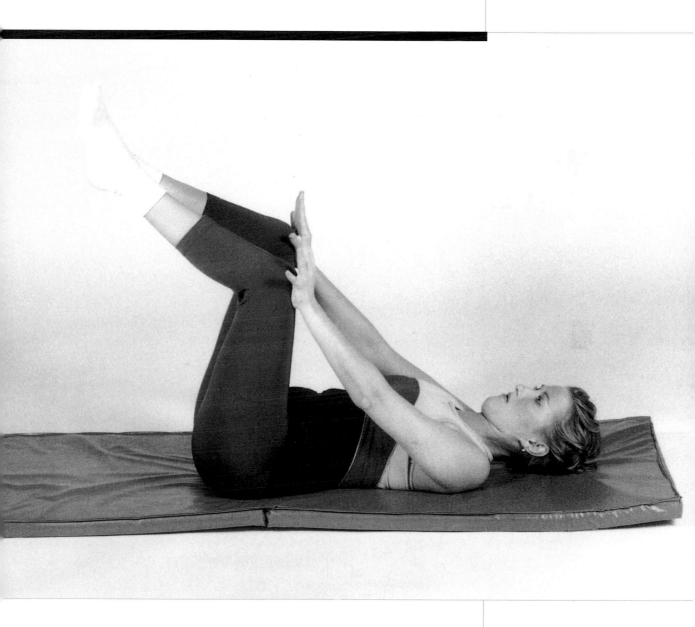

exercise **one**

FORM CHECK:

- Keep the back of your head on the mat as you tuck in your chin.
- Be sure to keep your shoulders on the mat for the full exercise.
- Your knees will lift slightly and your buttocks will tighten as you flatten your lower back into the mat.
- To really stretch your leg muscles, be sure to push the backs of your knees into the mat as you flex your feet.

THE PURPOSE This warm-up exercise targets six hot spots: the muscles of the neck, shoulders, upper and lower back, pelvic region and legs. The long stretch down the length of your body helps to alleviate spinal joint compression. This exercise gets to the core of muscle tension and relieves it.

START Lie on your back, legs flat, keeping your hands at your sides, palms up.

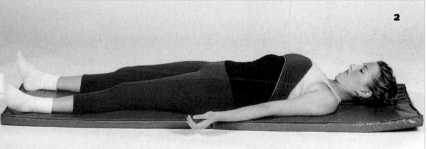

Leg Cramp Reliever

The Full Head-to-Toe Prep is an excellent way to alleviate or prevent nighttime leg and foot cramps. These painful spasms can be traced to tense muscles, which affect blood circulation in the back or legs, as well as compressed nerves, which compromise the flow of electrical signals from your nerves to your muscles. If you suffer from leg cramps, try performing ten repetitions of this movement before going to bed.

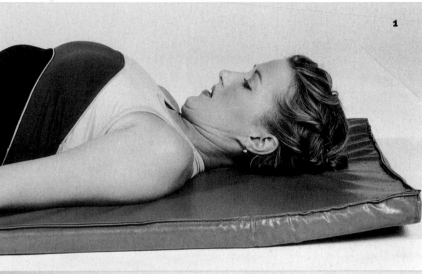

head-to-toe prep

THE MOVEMENT

■ **Neck retraction.**
Elongate the back of your neck by tucking your chin down toward your chest. Hold the position as you count out loud to six and then release it. [1

■ **Shoulder press-down.**
Push your shoulder blades together and down into the mat. Hold the position as you count out loud to six and then release it. [2

■ **Rib pull-down.**
Cough to pull your rib cage down, which contracts the oblique abdominal muscles. Hold the position as you count out loud to six and then release it.

■ **Pelvic tilt.**
Tilt your pubic bone toward your navel as you contract your abdominals and flatten your lower back into the mat. Hold the position as you count out loud to six and then release it. [3

■ **Knee press.**
With your legs extended as long as they can be, press the backs of your knees into the mat and flex your feet. Hold the position as you count out loud to six and then release it. [4

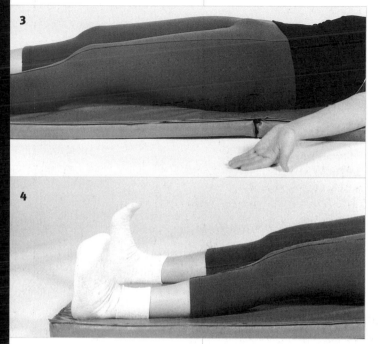

TIP:
You may feel some initial discomfort in the shoulder blades while you do the exercise. This should disappear as soon as you stop the exercise.

Full Head-to-Toe Prep
Put it all together: [5

■ Tuck in chin.

■ Open shoulders by pressing shoulder blades together.

■ Cough to pull rib cage down.

■ Tilt pubic bone as you contract your abdominals.

■ Straighten legs as you flex feet.

■ Hold tightly as you count out loud, this time for a count of twelve, and then release.

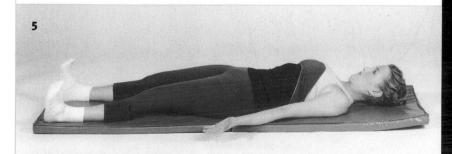

exercise **two**

THE PURPOSE   This terrific stretch hones in on a set of muscles that are usually ignored: the hardworking muscles that support the eyes. Many of us spend the majority of our working hours looking either downward or forward. This exercise reverses the strain by directing you to look upward and backward.

The Tongue Stretch also eases tension in the muscles of the face and jaw, alleviating headaches. So if you grind your teeth or have TMJ (temporomandibular joint disorder), this exercise will help you, too. One other benefit is cosmetic: The more you stick out your tongue, the more you will relax your facial muscles, which will minimize the folds in the skin of your face. If you want to, you can do the Tongue Stretch six times a day, and if you can't lie down to do it, you can do it just as effectively sitting at your desk.

START   Lie flat on your back, face relaxed, keeping your arms next to you on the mat, palms up.

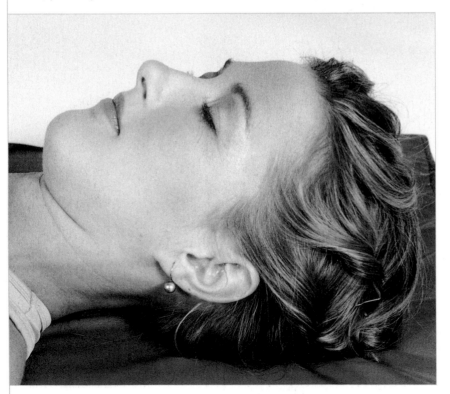

tongue stretch

Stretch the Vagus Nerve

If your physician has ruled out any serious pathology but you are still suffering from any of the following—difficulty swallowing, digestive problems such as heartburn, reflux and nausea, ringing in the ears or heart palpitations, the Tongue Stretch might be very helpful for you. The reason is that this exercise elongates the tissues surrounding the vagus nerve, also known as the "wandering nerve." The vagus nerve originates in the brain and makes its way through the front of the neck, then branches into the esophagus, heart and stomach. If you have any of the above symptoms and an organic cause cannot be found, it may be because the soft tissue surrounding your vagus nerve has become constricted and is in need of being stretched. This will free the nerve so it can deliver its signals fully and efficiently.

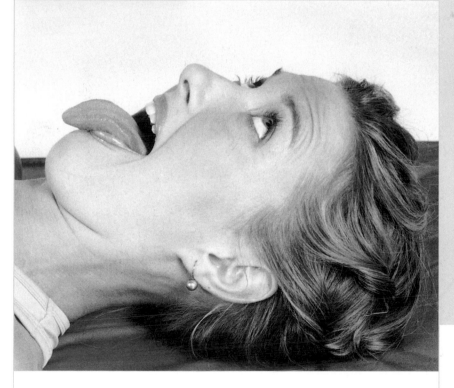

exercise **three**

THE PURPOSE This exercise creates a girdle of muscle to support the spine, giving you the support you need for daily activities as well as for sports. It also strengthens the abdominal zone and the hot spot pelvic area, where it enhances bladder control by strengthening pelvic floor muscles.

START Lie on your back with knees bent at a 90 degree angle and hands on your stomach. [**1**

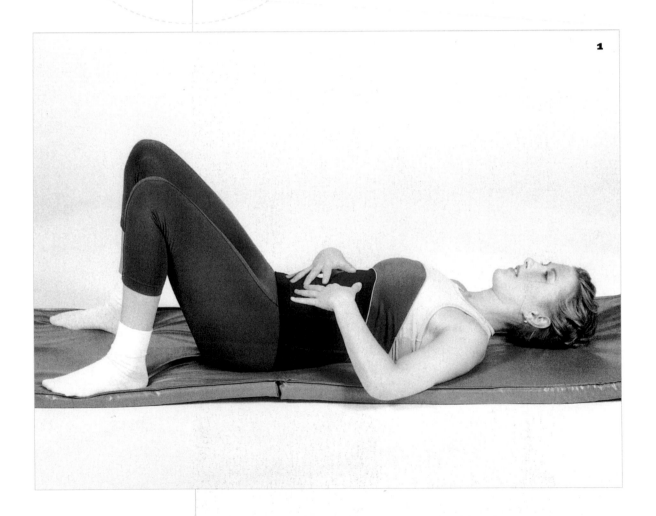

1

belly blaster

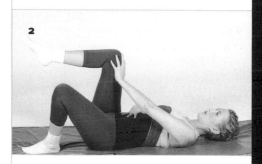

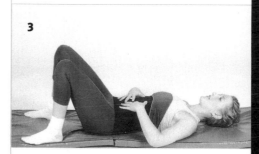

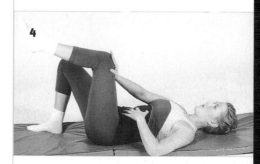

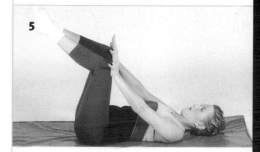

THE MOVEMENT

- Tilt your pelvis to press your lower back into the mat, elongate the back of your neck with your head resting on the mat and suck in your abdomen. Hold the position as you count out loud to six and then release it.

- Once again tilt your pelvis, elongate the back of your neck and contract your abdominals.

- Lift your right leg up with the knee bent. Keeping your back and shoulders on the mat, extend your left arm straight across your body until it reaches the right knee. Push your left hand against your right knee while the knee resists the pressure. Hold the position as you count out loud to six and then release it. [2

- Repeat three times and return to starting position. [3

- Switch to your left leg and right arm and perform the same exercise, repeating three times. [4

- Do the same exercise involving both legs simultaneously. Push your right hand against your right knee and your left hand against your left knee, while the knees resist the pressure from your hands. Hold the position as you count out loud to six and then release it. [5

- Repeat three times.

FORM CHECK:

- Make sure that your elbows are straight when you push against your knees.

- Keep head and shoulders on the mat. Press the hollow of your lower spine down into the mat as well.

exercise **four**

THE PURPOSE It's time to take a deep breath to replenish the oxygen you've used in the previous exercises. At the same time you'll be preparing yourself for the next exercise, because breathing deeply will allow you greater range of motion. And, taking this "break" will make you feel great.

START Lie on your stomach with your arms at your sides. Turn your head to one side.

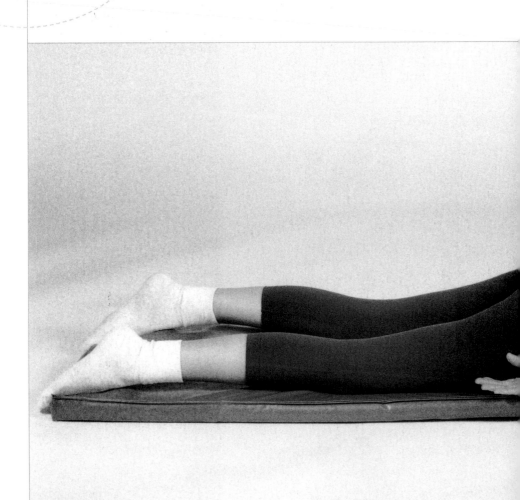

belly breath

THE MOVEMENT

- Take a long, slow breath through your nostrils, filling up your belly and your lungs as you count to four to yourself.
- Hold the breath for seven seconds.
- Exhale through your nose as you count out loud to eight.
- Turn your head to the opposite side and repeat.

TIPS:

- As you inhale, imagine the warm air flowing to all parts of your body.
- As you gently exhale, imagine the tension flowing out of all your muscles.

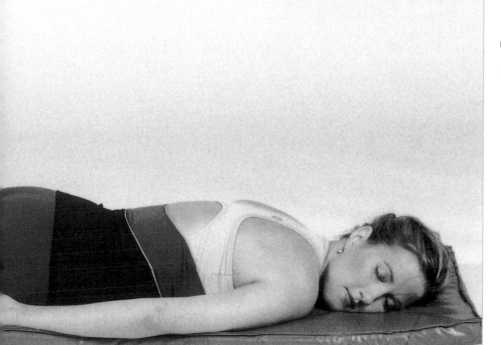

exercise **five**

FORM CHECK:

- As you begin your stretch, imagine your spine as a banana that you are slowly peeling from your neck, to midback, to lower back.

- Instead of tightening your buttocks as you lift off the mat, which limits the spinal extension, just press up with your arms into the range that is most comfortable. With each repetition, attempt to press up higher, keeping your buttocks relaxed.

- Keep your back relaxed and "flaccid." Don't hunch your shoulders together. Let your arms do the work.

- Try not to scrunch the muscles at the back of your neck together as you look up at the ceiling. Think about elongating the back of the neck at the same time that you are tilting it back, and pushing up and out from the chest.

THE PURPOSE I've included this classic yoga position for a very good reason: The series of movements increases your body's overall muscle flexibility as well as its core strength. Several hot spots are targeted. The muscles of the upper and lower back are relaxed, taking pressure off nerves and spinal disks. The hip-flexor muscles are elongated, further reducing pressure and tension on the lower back. At the same time, the muscles of the abdomen, neck and hips are gently stretched. By elongating soft tissue in the front of the body, the vagus nerve is lengthened, the rib cage is opened and your internal organs are given optimal space in which to function.

A whopping 90 percent of my patients respond to this graceful spinal-extension exercise, which either reduces or eliminates acute and chronic lower-back discomfort. The majority of my patients who suffer from herniated disks find this to be the only exercise they need to do to alleviate their pain.

START Lie on your stomach, facedown into the mat, the back of your neck elongated. Place your palms on the mat, at the sides of your shoulders. Keep the tops of your feet resting on the mat.

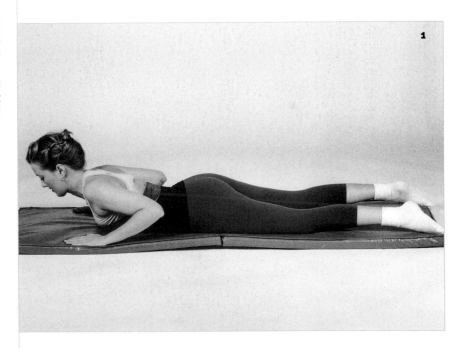

1

THE MOVEMENT

- Push up, tilting your head back slightly, in the sequence of forehead, nose and chin. [1

- Face forward as you rise, pushing up on your arms and opening your chest, keeping your pubic bone pushed into the mat while relaxing the buttocks as best you can. [2

- Slowly arch your spine backward, straightening, but not locking, your elbows.

- Roll your head back until you are looking straight up at the ceiling. [3

- Hold the position as you count out loud to three. Then descend slowly to the mat. [4

- Repeat six times.

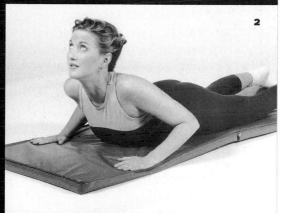

2

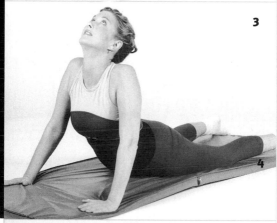

3

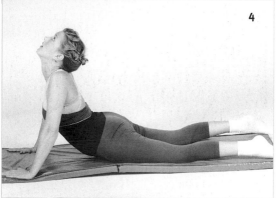

4

TIPS:

- If your lower back is very stiff, you won't be able to keep your pelvis on the mat. Don't worry about it. Simply raise your pelvis off the mat as you straighten your arms. As you become more limber and flexible through the lower back, you will be able to keep your pelvis on the mat.

- If you're unable to lift yourself by straightening your arms, do the backward stretch while propped up on your elbows, which should be close in to your chest.

- You may feel some discomfort or stiffness in your lower back, but this will diminish, and may be eliminated completely over time. With each repetition, you should feel a little more flexible.

exercise **six**

THE PURPOSE   This super two-part exercise delivers a double punch. The Butterfly stabilizes the muscles in the hot spots of the neck, shoulders and upper back. Doing the movements will strengthen your back as well as improve your posture.

Heel Beats, by concentrating on the hot spots in the lower back, knees and hips (as well as the inner thighs), builds leg power. Everything from going down steps to running to playing sports will be easier to do.

Even more important, every time you do the Butterfly/Heel Beats combination, you are helping to prevent osteoporosis. As the movements force back muscles to pull on vertebrae, they promote the building of new bone cells. The movements also help align your spine, which allows proper weight bearing throughout the column of vertebrae.

BUTTERFLY

START   Lie on your stomach with your forehead resting on the mat. Keep your arms at your sides, palms facing upward. [**1**

FORM CHECK:

- Your head should not be higher or lower than your shoulders. Keep your ears aligned with your shoulders and your face parallel to the floor, looking down.

- Pinch your shoulder blades together as much as possible.

- Don't lift your legs off the mat.

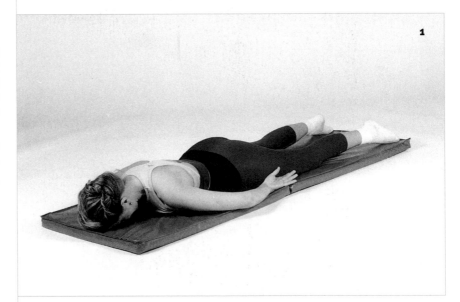

1

butterfly/heel beats combo

THE MOVEMENT

- Contract your abdominal muscles. Push your pubic bone into the mat and then squeeze your shoulder blades together. Slowly raise your chest off the mat as high as possible by pinching your shoulder blades together. At the same time, raise your arms to the level of your buttocks. [2

- Keep the back of your neck elongated, chin slightly tucked in, with eyes focused downward. [3

- Hold the position as you count out loud to six and then release it.

- Return to the starting position and then perform Heel Beats (following).

TIP:

- If you're unable to lift your chest off the mat, just squeeze your shoulder blades together and complete the exercise.

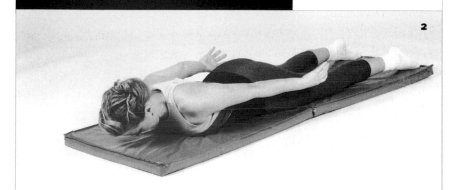

2

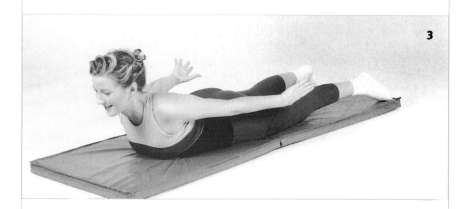

3

HEEL BEATS

START Lie on your stomach with the backs of your hands creating a pillow for your forehead and press your pubic bone into the mat by recruiting your abdominal muscles. [1

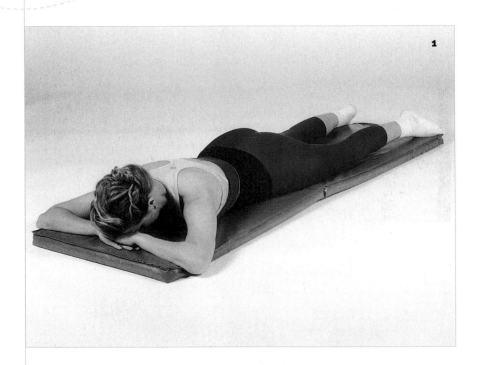

1

butterfly/heel beats combo

THE MOVEMENT

- Lift your legs off the mat to buttock level, a little wider than shoulder-width apart. [2

- Click your heels together quickly, then back to shoulder-width apart, with toes turned outward. Repeat this in-out motion as many times as you can while counting out loud to twenty. [3

- Return your legs to the mat and perform a Butterfly.

  Perform another twenty-count Heel Beats and finish with a Butterfly, for a total of three Butterflies and two Heel Beats.

FORM CHECK:

- Keep your face down, head parallel to the floor.

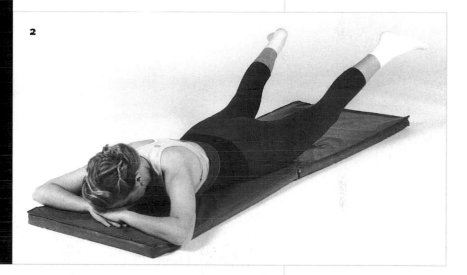

2

TIPS:

- If you can't lift your legs off the mat, tighten your buttocks and slide your legs in and out along the mat for the allotted time.

- If you feel any discomfort in your lower back, push your pubic bone farther into the mat.

- If discomfort continues, put a pillow under your stomach and try to complete the exercise.

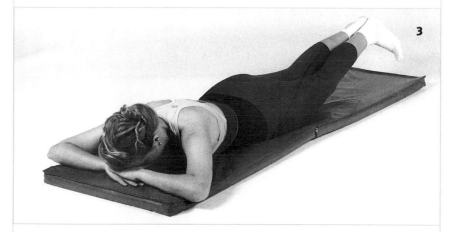

3

exercise **seven**

THE PURPOSE   Building up the muscles of the hot spot pelvic area is very important, since the pelvis is the foundation of the whole spine and the place where the upper and lower body come together. Stabilizing the pelvis means that sitting, rising, walking, running—any motion that requires the legs to move—will all be easier and less tiring.

The first two parts of the exercise warm up pelvic muscles and stretch nerves as they work the hamstrings, the long muscles that run from the hip, down the back of the thigh, to the knee. They also work the muscles around the hips and the lower back, and the quadriceps in the thighs, as well as the abdominals. The third part strengthens the upper and lower parts of the legs and tones the buttocks.

All three parts of the exercise are performed on one side before switching to the other.

PART ONE: HAMSTRING SIDE KICK

START   Lie on your left side, propped on your left elbow. Raise your upper body, contract your abdominal muscles and support your weight on the left forearm, which is flat on the mat. Keep your left fist on the mat as well. Keep your legs straight, one on top of the other, at a 45 degree angle from your torso.

Place your right palm on the mat in front of you, your right forearm against your tightened abdomen, with the elbow pressed against the pelvic bone to eliminate the tendency to roll backward.

three-part pelvic stabilizer

THE MOVEMENT

- Lift your right leg three inches. [1
- Gently kick forward as far as possible with foot flexed, maintaining contact of the right elbow with the pelvis. [2
- Return to the starting position.
- Repeat six times as you count out loud to six.

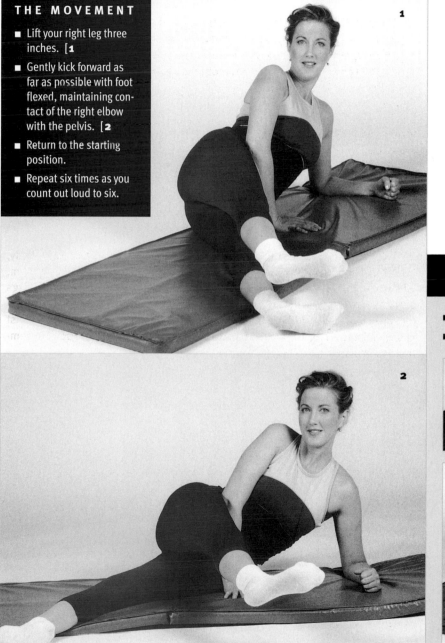

1

2

Make Sure You Don't:

- Slump forward.
- Roll back.

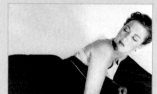

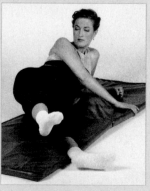

exercise **seven**

CONT.

PART TWO: GLUTEAL TONER

START Lying on your left side in the starting position, flex your right foot and lift your right leg three inches. [**1**

THE MOVEMENT

- Kick your leg backward. [**2**
- Return to the starting position.
- Repeat six times as you count out loud to six.

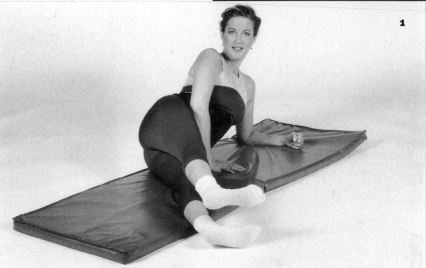

Make Sure You Don't:

Arch your back by kicking your leg too far behind you.

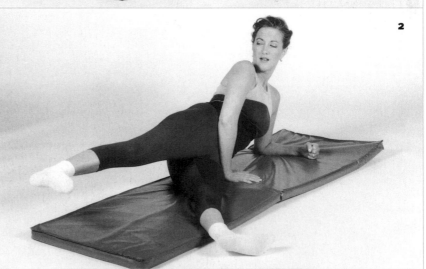

PART THREE:
FOOT CIRCLES

START Lie on your left side in the starting position. [1

THE MOVEMENT

- Rotate your right leg so toes are flexed toward ceiling, and lift the leg three inches, maintaining contact of the right elbow against the pelvis. [2
- Circle your leg clockwise, clicking your right heel against your left foot six times as you count out loud to six. Then circle counterclockwise six times as you count out loud to six.
- Repeat all three exercises on the opposite leg.

FORM CHECK:

- It's important to keep your top forearm braced against the pelvis. This constant contact ensures that you remain in the proper position, preventing you from rolling backward.

TIPS:

- If you're unable to lift your leg to the prescribed height, lift it as high as you're able.
- If you can't continue for the allotted number of repetitions, take a brief rest and then continue.
- If you are unable to keep your torso elevated, lie on your side with your head resting on your outstretched arm.

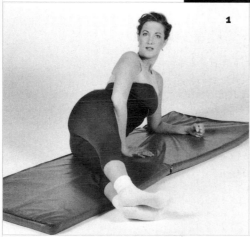

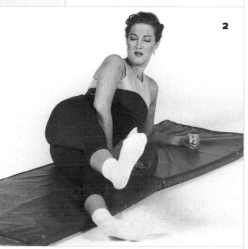

exercise **eight**

THE PURPOSE   This multi-part exercise provides alternating contraction and relaxation in order to gradually stretch even the tightest hamstring muscles—the long muscles on the back of the thighs. Increasing hamstring flexibility will help protect you from back problems—or relieve any discomfort you already have.

The first two movements elongate the hamstring muscles and give your hot spot muscles in the lower back and hips additional flexibility. The third part stretches the soft tissue around the sciatic nerve, which is the nerve that runs all the way from the spine down the length of both legs and supplies the legs with sensory and motor control. If that tissue gets shortened, it can entrap the sciatic nerve and interfere with its ability to deliver its signals. Nighttime leg cramps can also stem from an entrapped sciatic nerve.

The last movement strengthens the quadriceps, the muscles on the front of the thighs, which are one of the body's largest and most powerful muscle groups. You need strong quadriceps to balance the power of the hamstrings.

It's important to remember that each of the movements is a continuation of the one before it, so the sequence should flow seamlessly from start to finish. If you find that you can't straighten your leg fully during the exercise, just extend your leg as much as you comfortably can.

All four parts of the exercise are performed on one side before switching to the other.

PART ONE: KNEE TO CHEST STRETCH

START   Lie on your back with knees bent and feet flat on the mat. Arms are by your sides, palms down. [**1**

FORM CHECK:

- Keep your shoulders down on the mat and your chin tucked in, which helps elongate your neck.

- Be sure to release the knee between each repetition of the stretch. This reduces the muscle tension, allowing the hamstring a chance to stretch farther each time.

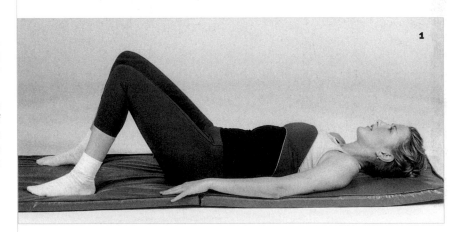

1

four-part progressive hamstring stretch

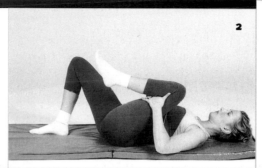

2

TIP:

- Take your thigh back as far as you can while still keeping your back flat on the floor. You may feel some discomfort but it will disappear as you become more flexible.

THE MOVEMENT

- Contract your abdominal muscles, elongate the back of your neck and press your lower back into the mat. *You will maintain this contraction and elongation through all four parts of the exercise.*

- Wrap your hands behind your left thigh and gently pull the left knee toward your chest. [2

- Hold the position as you count out loud to six and then release it.

- Slowly slide your right leg down along the mat as you release your left thigh to a 90 degree angle. [3

- Gently pull the left thigh back to your chest. Hold the position as you count out loud to six and then release it. [4

- Repeat the stretch three times while your right leg remains flat on the mat. Release the left thigh to a 90 degree angle in preparation for the next exercise. [5

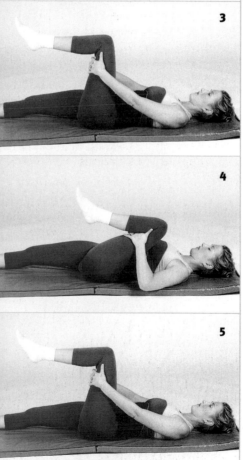

3

4

5

exercise **eight**
CONT.

PART TWO:
**STRAIGHT-LEG
PRESSURE-ON,
PRESSURE-OFF
HAMSTRING STRETCH**

THE MOVEMENT

- Straighten your left leg as much as you can with both hands behind the knee, while the right leg remains flat on the floor. [**1**
- Bend your knee so your shin drops to a horizontal position. [**2**
- Return the leg to the vertical position. Repeat six times as you count out loud to six.
- End with your leg straight up in preparation for the next exercise. [**3**

FORM CHECK:

- Be sure your shoulders are kept on the mat.
- Keep your abdominal muscles tightened so that your lower back remains in contact with the mat at all times. If you feel strain in your back, bending the working leg slightly will help.

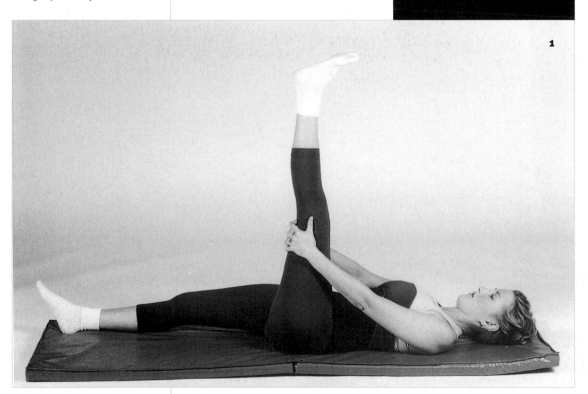

1

2

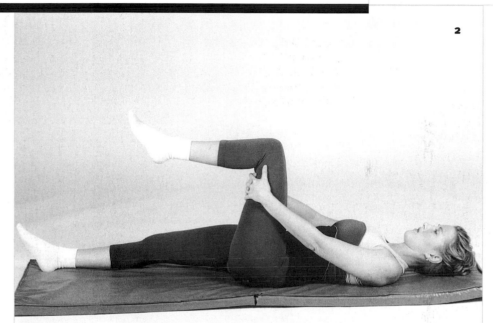

3

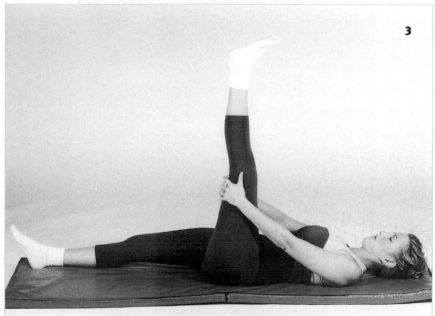

exercise **eight**

**PART THREE:
ANKLE PUMP**

THE MOVEMENT

- Flex and release your foot six times as you count out loud to six. [**1**
- Finish with your leg straight up and foot flexed, which will take you into the next exercise. [**2**

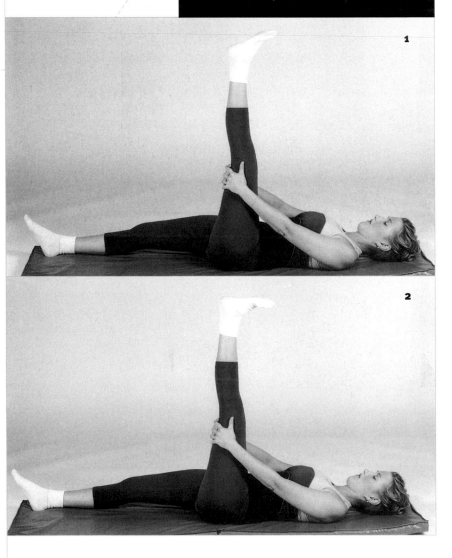

FORM CHECK:

- Be sure to contract your abdominals as you perform the exercise so that your lower back presses into the mat.
- Keep your shoulders on the mat to help maintain proper alignment. Place a pillow under your head if you cannot keep your shoulders down otherwise.

TIP:

- You may feel some discomfort behind your knee or in your hamstring as you perform the exercise. This will disappear as you gradually become more flexible.

four-part progressive hamstring stretch

THE MOVEMENT

- Lower your arms and brace them by your sides, palms down. [1

- Press your back into the mat, maximally tighten your buttocks and left thigh and keep your foot flexed. Hold the position as you count out loud to six.

- Keeping the contraction in all your muscles, slowly lower your leg, as you count out loud to six, until it comes to rest on the mat. [2, [3

- Repeat all four exercises with your right leg.

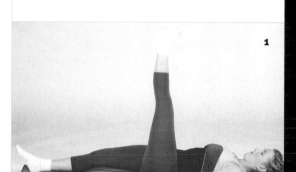

1

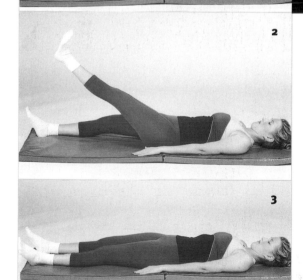

2

3

TIPS:

- Make sure to keep your back pressed into the mat, especially when lowering the leg.

- If you can't keep your back pressed into the mat, place both hands under your buttocks for support.

exercise **nine**

THE PURPOSE   This exercise stretches the muscles and soft tissue throughout the lower-back hot-spot area. Next, it opens up the foramina, which are the bony openings between the vertebrae, where the nerve roots exit the spinal cord. This allows for more complete nerve firing. Finally, it stretches the muscles of your hip hot spots.

The result of all these actions is that nerve compression in the spine will be eased. Therefore, you'll be able to sit, bend and stand with a lot more comfort and endurance. In short, you'll have greater mobility.

START   Lie on your back with knees bent, feet flat on the mat, with the palms of your hands resting on your thighs. Elongate your neck, tuck in your chin and make sure your shoulders are on the mat. Keep your abdominal muscles tightened and your lower back pressed down. [**1**

FORM CHECK:

- Shoulders remain on the mat the entire time.
- Don't rock and roll your spine.

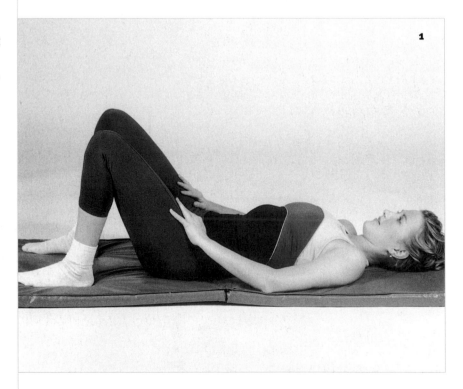

1

double knees to chest

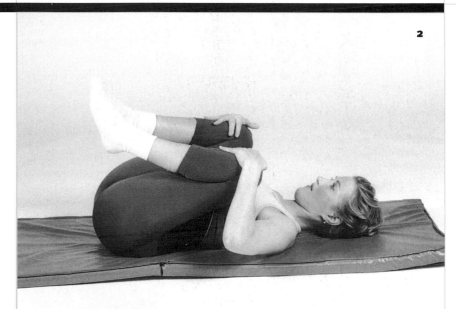

2

TIP:

- Be sure to breathe deeply. This will make it easier to bring your knees closer to your chest.

THE MOVEMENT

- Lift your knees and pull them back toward your chest. [2
- Hold the position as you count out loud to six and then release knees to the starting position. [3
- Repeat three times.

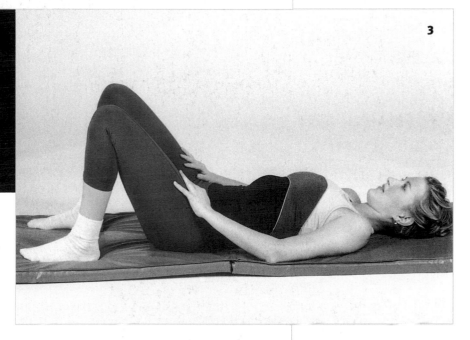

3

exercise **ten**

THE PURPOSE   This exercise compensates for the asymmetry in the hips, pelvis and lower-back muscles, which is caused by favoring muscles on one side of the body over another. For instance, most women prefer to cross one leg, say, the left over the right, and not the other way around. Over time, the muscles of the uncrossed leg become shortened. Favoring one side of the body while doing any regular activities—playing tennis or golf, or even "phone hugging" on your preferred shoulder—can cause muscle shortening.

This movement also stretches the muscles in the chest, shoulders and neck as your head tilts to counteract the shift in your pelvis.

START   Lie on your back with your head looking up at the ceiling. Bent knees are together, ankles are touching and feet are flat on the mat. Keep your arms straight out to the sides at shoulder height, so your body forms the letter T. Elongate your neck and make sure your shoulders are on the mat. Contract your abdominal muscles and press your lower back into the mat. [**1**

FORM CHECK:

- Be sure to keep your shoulders on the mat.

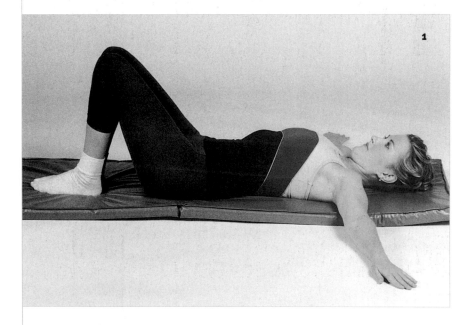

1

lying spinal twist

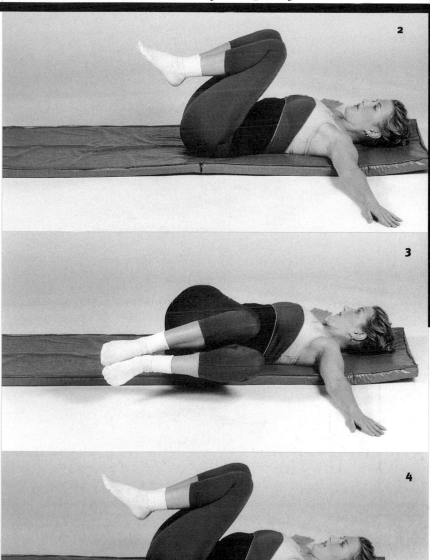

2

3

4

THE MOVEMENT

- Gradually lift the knees to your chest. [2
- Slowly drop both legs to the left side. [3
- Slowly rotate your head to the right side, keeping both shoulders flat on the mat.
- Hold the position as you count out loud to six and then pull your knees back to your chest. [4
- Repeat on the opposite side.
- Perform a total of four twists, two for each side.

TIP:

- As you gain flexibility, both sides of your body will feel equally relaxed.

exercise **eleven**

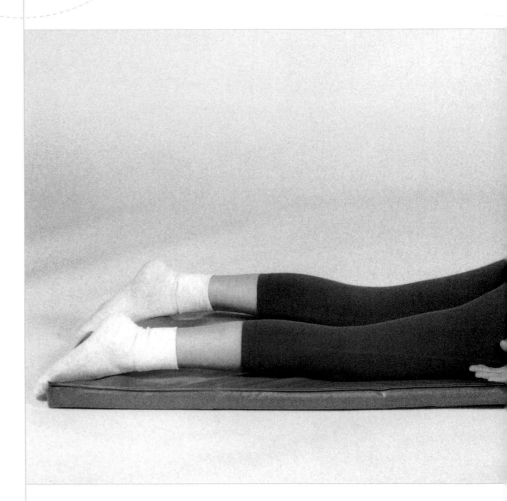

belly breath

THE MOVEMENT

- Take a long, slow breath through your nostrils, filling up your belly and your lungs as you count to four to yourself.
- Hold the breath for seven seconds.
- Exhale through your nose as you count out loud to eight.
- Turn your head to the opposite side and repeat.

TIPS:

- As you inhale, imagine the warm air flowing to all parts of your body.
- As you gently exhale, imagine the tension flowing out of all your muscles.

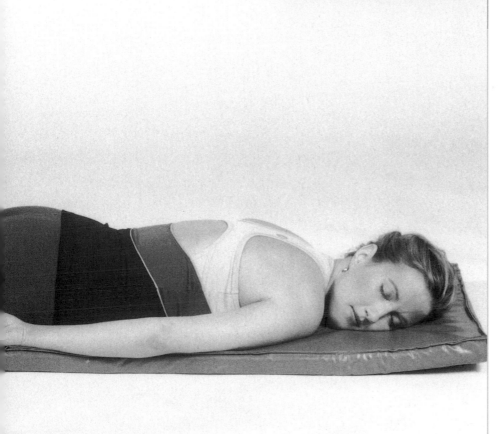

exercise **twelve**

THE PURPOSE   This exercise bolsters coordination between the arms and legs. Synchronizing the action of the extremities has an immediate effect: improved balance and a heightened sense of stability. This, in turn, will give you greater grace and ease of movement. Also, this full-body strengthening gives the upper and lower muscles a thorough lengthening by extending them simultaneously in opposite directions.

START   Lie on your stomach with your forehead resting on the mat and your arms, extended palms down, in front of your head. Elongate the back of your neck and tighten your abdominals as you press your pubic bone into the mat. [**1**

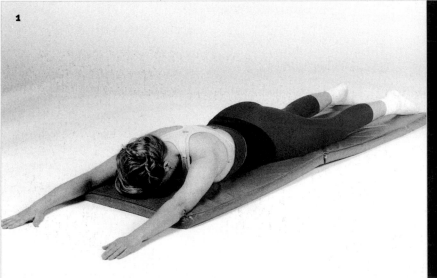

1

THE MOVEMENT

- Extend your right arm in front of you as far as possible and lift it three to six inches, while simultaneously raising your left leg three to six inches, with the toes pointed back as far as possible. [**2**
- Hold the position as you count out loud to six. Then release and return to the starting position. [**3**
- Repeat with the opposite arm and leg.
- Repeat three times.

FORM CHECK:

- Keep your head facing down, and the back of the neck long and straight.
- Be sure to keep your pubic bone pressed into the mat for spinal stability.

cross extension

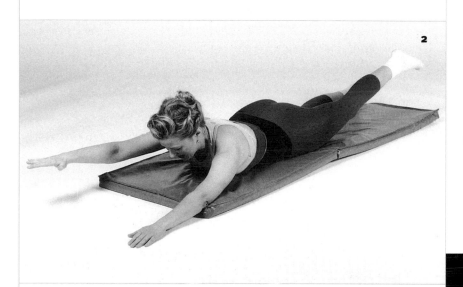

2

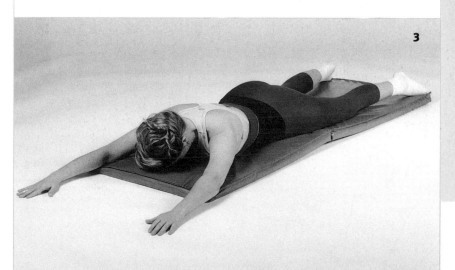

3

TIPS:

- Think of reaching forward with your hand as far as you can, at the same time reaching back with your foot as far as you can. Feel your body growing longer.
- If you can't lift a leg, just extend it and stretch your toes as far back as possible.

Make Sure You Don't:

- Lift your leg too high.
- Lift your arm too high.

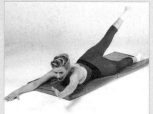

exercise **thirteen**

FORM CHECK:

- As you begin your stretch, imagine your spine as a banana that you are slowly peeling from your neck, to midback, to lower back.

- Instead of tightening your buttocks as you lift off the mat, which limits the spinal extension, just press up with your arms into the range that is most comfortable. With each repetition, attempt to press up higher, keeping your buttocks relaxed.

- Keep your back relaxed and "flaccid." Don't hunch your shoulders together. Let your arms do the work.

- Try not to scrunch the muscles at the back of your neck together as you look up at the ceiling. Think about elongating the back of the neck at the same time that you are tilting it back, and pushing up and out from the chest.

I have included another Cobra near the end of the Core Foundation because it gently relaxes all the muscles you've just exerted. If you had trouble keeping your pelvis on the mat while performing the previous set of Cobras, see how much more flexible you are during this round.

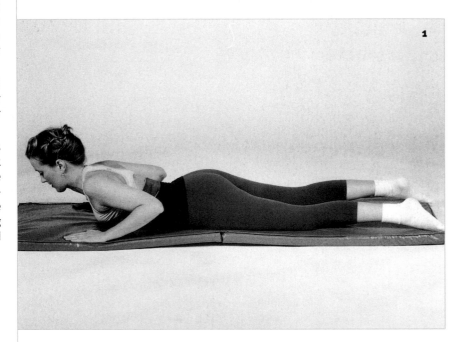

1

the cobra

THE MOVEMENT

- Push up, tilting your head back slightly, in the sequence of forehead, nose and chin. [1
- Face forward as you rise, pushing up on your arms and opening your chest, keeping your pubic bone pushed into the mat while relaxing the buttocks as best you can. [2
- Slowly arch your spine backward, straightening, but not locking, your elbows.
- Roll your head back until you are looking straight up at the ceiling. [3
- Hold the position as you count out loud to three. Then descend slowly to the mat. [4
- Repeat six times.

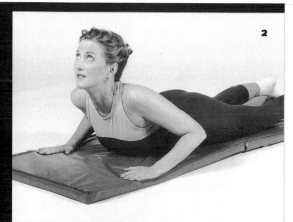

2

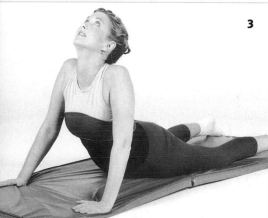

3

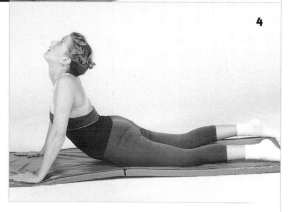

4

TIPS:

- If your lower back is very stiff, you won't be able to keep your pelvis on the mat. Don't worry about it. Simply raise your pelvis off the mat as you straighten your arms. As you become more limber and flexible through the lower back, you will be able to keep your pelvis on the mat.

- If you're unable to lift yourself by straightening your arms, do the backward stretch while propped up on your elbows, which should be close in to your chest.

- You may feel some discomfort or stiffness in your lower back, but this will diminish, and may be eliminated completely over time. With each repetition, you should feel a little more flexible.

exercise **fourteen**

This exercise finishes out the Core Foundation by helping you to relax all of your muscles with deep, rhythmical breathing.

Repeat the directions in Exercise #4.

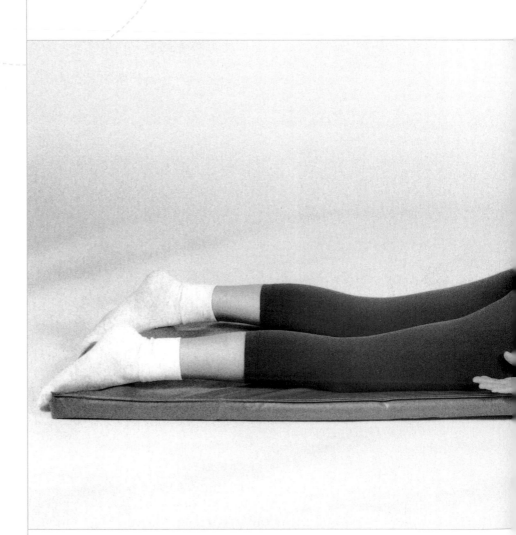

belly breath finale

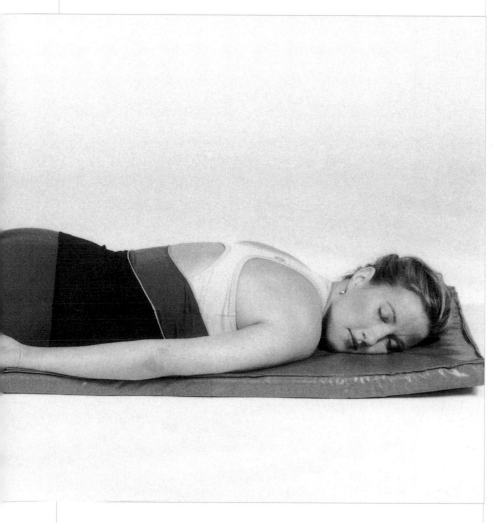

CONGRATULATIONS!
You've completed the Core Foundation, the basis of looking and feeling as good as you possibly can.

the core foundation

1. Head-to-Toe Prep

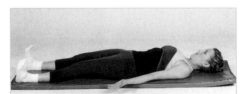

2. Tongue Stretch

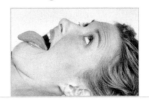

3. Belly Blaster

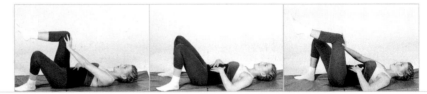

4. Belly Breath

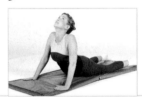

5. The Cobra

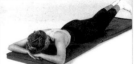

6. Butterfly/Heel Beats Combo

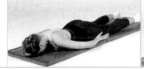 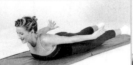 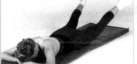 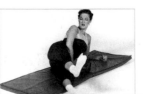

7. Three-Part Pelvic Stabilizer

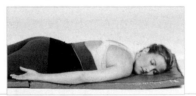 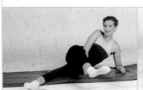 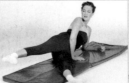

8. Four-Part Progressive Hamstring Stretch

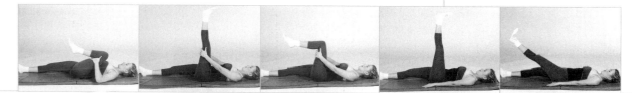

9. Double Knees to Chest

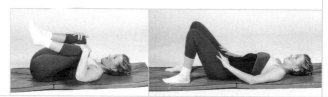

10. Lying Spinal Twist   **11.** Belly Breath

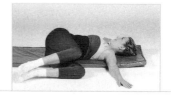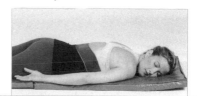

12. Cross Extension

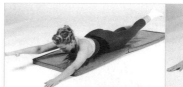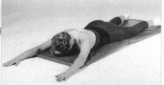

13. The Cobra   **14.** Belly Breath Finale

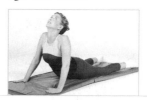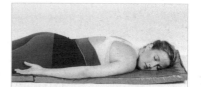

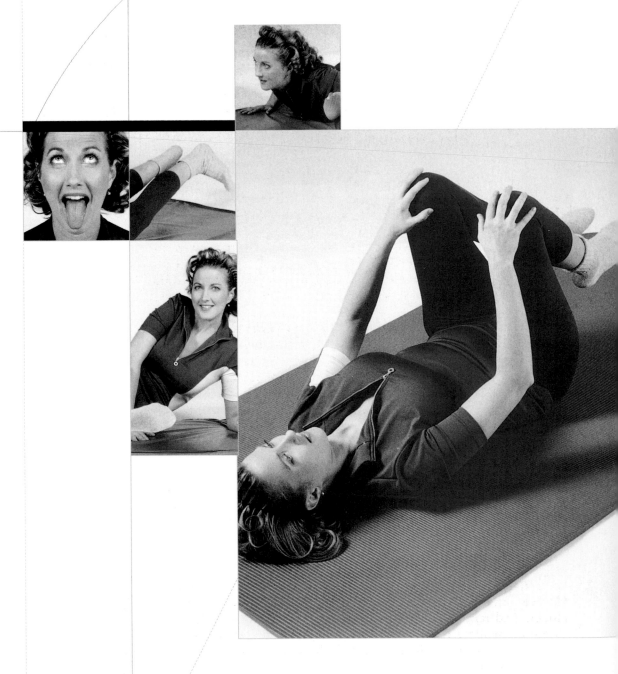

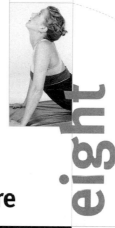

The Intermediate Core

After you do the Core Foundation for three weeks you can opt to move on to the more challenging Intermediate Core. You'll know you are ready when you feel strong and flexible and find the Core Foundation exercises easier to do.

In this Core Program, your extremities work in new, more demanding ways. Thanks to the isometric contractions of the Core Foundation you are ready to handle more isotonic movements, because your muscles are now strong enough to keep your joints aligned as you do these exercises.

In this new Core, I've included some movements you've mastered—their effects only increase over time—along with six new exercises. The combination of old and new exercises will continue to increase your strength, your stability, your balance and your ease of movement. One exercise from the Foundation—the Three-Part Pelvic Stabilizer—takes on a new dimension with the addition of ankle weights, which will tone your legs even more. I've even added a special set of exercises that concentrate on smoothing facial muscles. Consider it facial fitness!

You'll notice that some of the new exercises have more than six reps. Because these exercises are more intense and require more time, they create an even greater body toning effect. However, if there are days when you are extra tired and don't feel up to doing the Intermediate Core, feel free to go back and do the Core Foundation.

Before you begin your exercises, place your ankle weights—one pound if you're just beginning, or two pounds if you've worked up to that—near your mat so you'll have them handy when you need them. And remember: Unless otherwise stated, the exercises that are done while lying on your back are performed with your chin retracted, your abdominal muscles hollowed out and your pelvis slightly tilted.

the intermediate core

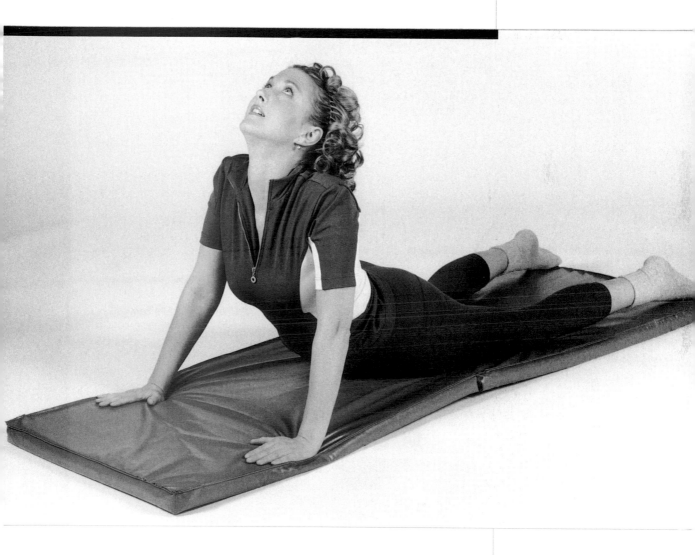

exercise **one**

FORM CHECK:

- Keep the back of your head on the mat as you tuck your chin.
- Be sure to keep your shoulders on the mat for the full exercise.
- Your knees will lift slightly and your buttocks will tighten as you flatten your lower back into the mat.
- To really stretch your leg muscles, be sure to push the backs of your knees into the mat as you flex your feet.

THE PURPOSE Preparing your body for the other movements in the program is crucial. Since it's such a terrific full-body stretch, I begin by having you repeat the Head-to-Toe Prep you've already mastered in the Core Foundation. You'll be warming and stretching your muscles as you keep improving your alignment.

START Lie on your back, legs flat, keeping your hands at your sides, palms up. [**1**

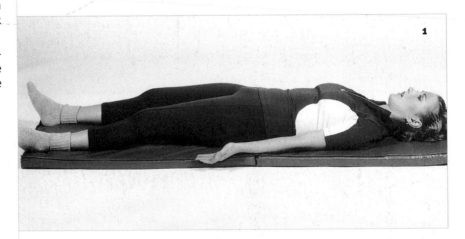

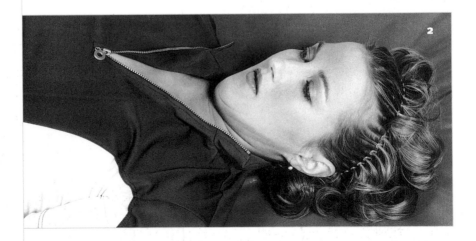

head-to-toe prep

THE MOVEMENT

■ **Neck retraction.**
Elongate the back of your neck by tucking your chin down toward your chest. Hold the position as you count out loud to six and then release It. [2

■ **Shoulder press-down.**
Push your shoulder blades together and down into the mat. Hold the position as you count out loud to six and then release it. [3

■ **Rib pull-down.**
Cough to pull your rib cage down, which contracts the oblique abdominal muscles. Hold the position as you count out loud to six and then release it.

■ **Pelvic tilt.**
Tilt your pubic bone toward your navel as you contract your abdominals and flatten your lower back into the mat. Hold the position as you count out loud to six and then release it.

■ **Knee press.**
With your legs extended as long as they can be, press the backs of your knees into the mat and flex your feet. Hold the position as you count out loud to six and then release it. [4

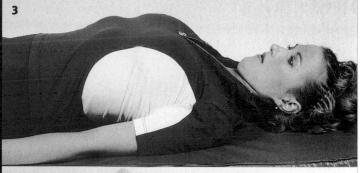

3

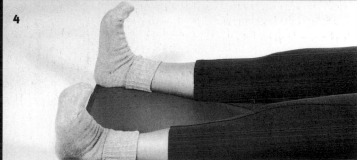

4

TIP:
You may feel some initial discomfort in the shoulder blades while you do the exercise. This should disappear as soon as you stop the exercise.

Full Head-to-Toe Prep [5
Put it all together:

■ Tuck in chin.

■ Open shoulders by pressing shoulder blades together.

■ Cough to pull rib cage down.

■ Tilt pubic bone as you contract your abdominals.

■ Press knees down as you flex feet.

■ Hold tightly as you count out loud, this time for a count of twelve, and then slowly release.

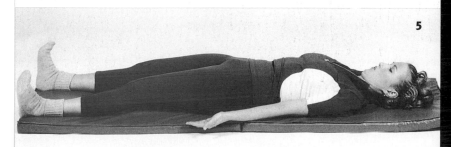

5

exercise **two**

THE PURPOSE   Dead Bugs work abdominal muscles by using an isometric contraction and then adding moving arms and legs as leverage against those muscles. The strengthening of the abdominal zone enables you to reach, carry or lift in the easiest, most effective way.

Doing this set of movements also works your arms and legs and helps cool one of the hot spots—the pelvic region, specifically the muscles of the pelvic floor. These are the muscles that hold the pubic bone and tailbone in place. The beauty of this exercise is that it doesn't exert too much pressure on the pelvic floor. Doing other abdominal-targeted muscles like sit-ups or curl-ups can cause the bladder and uterus to press on the pelvic floor, which may result in urinary incontinence. Since the pelvic floor muscles of women tend to lose strength as time goes on—as all muscles do if not exercised—the last thing we want to do is weaken them further. What we need to do is build them up. That is exactly what Dead Bugs does—strengthening the muscles that support the bladder, uterus and rectum. Toning the pelvic floor muscles provides an incredible spectrum of benefits: prevention of urinary incontinence problems, easier elimination, greater sexual enjoyment and quicker, easier childbirth. And if that isn't enough, consider this: Over time, doing Dead Bugs will give you a flatter silhouette by minimizing any "belly bulge." (Crunches, on the other hand, will do only one thing: help you get out of bed.)

START   Lie on your back with your knees bent and your feet flat on the mat. Keep your arms bent with the palms on your abdomen. Keep the back of your neck elongated with the chin tucked, and the small of your back pressed into the mat to maintain proper alignment and stabilize your back. **[1**

FORM CHECK:

- Don't bend your elbows—keep them locked—when you bring them back behind your head.

- Be sure to keep your shoulders on the mat.

- If you feel that your torso is moving from side to side, it means that you are not keeping your abdominal muscles contracted.

- Press your back to the mat to maintain your stable position.

- Be sure to keep your thumbs pointed toward the ceiling—as if you were hitchhiking. This form prevents impingement in your shoulders.

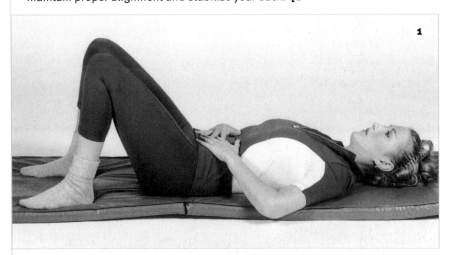

1

dead bugs

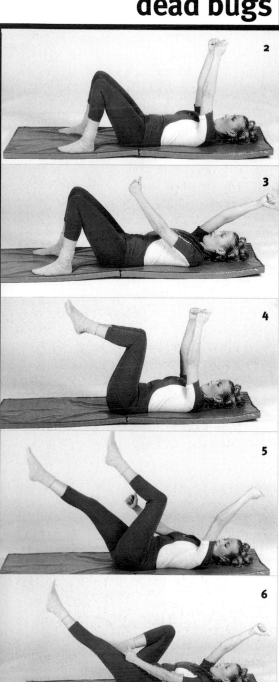

THE MOVEMENT

- Cough to recruit your upper abdominal and oblique muscles. Bring your arms straight up toward the ceiling, with your thumbs pointing up. [2
- While holding your abdominal contraction as tightly as possible, alternate extending your arms over your head as many times as you can as you count out loud to thirty. [3
- Contract your abdominal muscles. Keep both arms raised overhead. Now lift both knees toward your chest. [4
- Keeping your back flat against the mat, push your right leg out, then your left, alternating this gentle bicycling motion as many times as you can as you count out loud to thirty. [5
- Contract your abdominal muscles. Combine the arm and leg motions so that when one leg moves toward your chest, the arm on the same side is reaching over your head. Do as many alternating movements as you can as you count out loud to sixty. [6

TIPS:

- To properly recruit your abdominal muscles, Imagine that a zipper runs from your pubic bone to the lower portion of your rib cage and then pull it all the way up, as if zippering yourself in.
- Raise your legs away from your torso only as far as you can while still keeping your lower back pressed into the mat. If your back begins to lift off the mat, your abdominals are no longer engaged and you risk straining your back.
- If you can't maintain the pace for the allotted time because your abdominal muscles are fatiguing, stop moving your legs but continue alternating with your arms. If it's still too difficult, lower your legs and keep your arms moving.

exercise **three**

THE PURPOSE   After the exertion of Dead Bugs, you'll find doing this exercise twice as restorative as usual.

START   Lie on your stomach with your arms at your sides. Turn your head to one side.

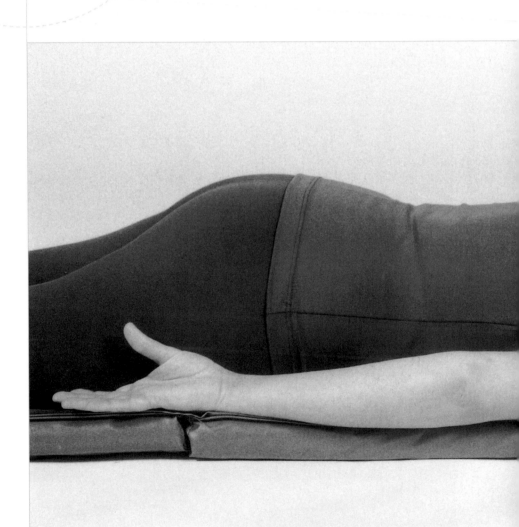

belly breath

THE MOVEMENT

- Take a long, slow breath through your nostrils, filling up your belly and your lungs as you silently count to four.
- Hold the breath for seven seconds.
- Exhale through your nose as you count out loud to eight.
- Turn your head to the opposite side and repeat.

TIPS:

- As you inhale, imagine the warm air flowing to all parts of your body.
- As you gently exhale, imagine the tension flowing out of all your muscles.

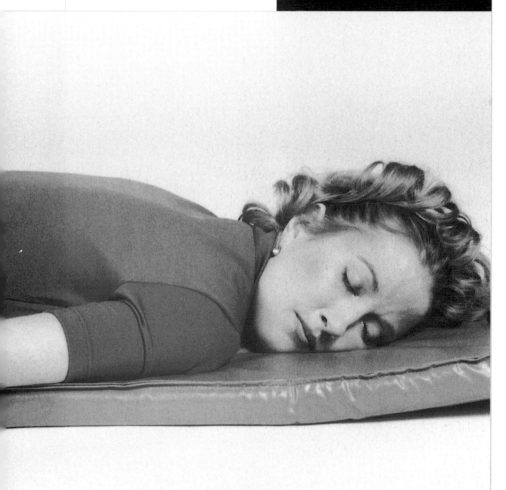

137

exercise **four**

FORM CHECK:

- As you begin your stretch, imagine your spine as a banana that you are slowly peeling from your neck, mid-back, then lower back.

- Instead of tightening your buttocks as you lift off the mat, which limits the spinal extension, just press up with your arms into the range that is most comfortable. With each repetition, attempt to press up higher, keeping your buttocks relaxed.

- Keep your back relaxed and "flaccid." Don't hunch your shoulders together. Let your arms do the work.

- Try not to scrunch the muscles at the back of your neck together as you look up at the ceiling. Think about elongating the back of the neck at the same time that you are tilting it back, and pushing up and out from the chest.

THE PURPOSE　The Cobra provides such a wide spectrum of benefits to the body—increasing its flexibility and strength and relieving the tension on several of your hot spots—that I'm repeating it in the Intermediate Core. And it's also worth repeating that a whopping 90 percent of my patients respond to this graceful spinal extension exercise, which either reduces or eliminates acute and chronic lower back discomfort. The majority of my patients who suffer from herniated disks find this to be the only exercise they need to do to alleviate their pain.

START　Lie on your stomach, facedown into the mat, the back of your neck elongated. Place your palms on the mat, at the sides of your shoulders. Keep the tops of your feet resting on the mat.

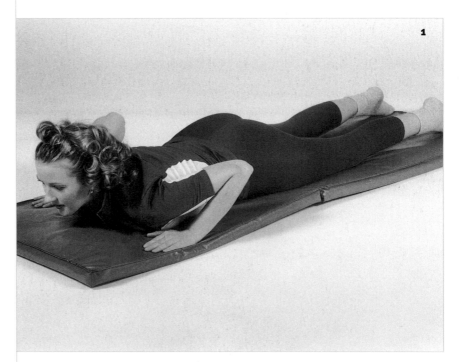

1

the cobra

THE MOVEMENT

- Push up, tilting your head back slightly, in the sequence of forehead, nose and chin. [1

- Face forward as you rise, pushing up on your arms and opening your chest, keeping your pubic bone pushed into the mat while relaxing the buttocks as best you can. [2

- Slowly arch your spine backward, straightening, but not locking, your elbows.

- Roll your head back until you are looking straight up at the ceiling. [3

- Hold the position as you count out loud to three and then descend slowly to the mat. [4

- Repeat six times.

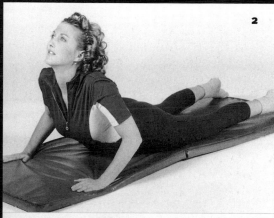

2

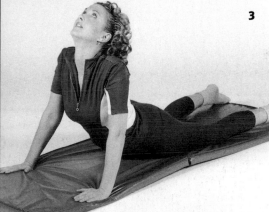

3

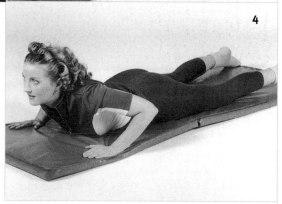

4

TIP:

- Even though you are familiar with the Cobra from the Core Foundation, you may still experience some stiffness on the initial press-up. But after each repetition, you should feel greater flexibility in your spine.

- If your lower back is very stiff, you won't be able to keep your pelvis on the mat. Don't worry about it. Simply raise your pelvis off the mat as you straighten your arms. As you become more limber and flexible through the lower back, you will be able to keep your pelvis on the mat.

- If you're unable to lift yourself by straightening your arms, do the backward stretch while propped up on your elbows, which should be close in to your chest.

exercise **five**

FORM CHECK:

- Your head should not be higher or lower than your shoulders. Keep your ears aligned with your shoulders and your face parallel to the floor, looking down.
- Don't lift your legs off the mat.
- If you can't do this variation, go back to the Core Foundation Butterfly on page 100 and then try this again after a week.

THE PURPOSE   This variation of the Core Foundation exercise intensifies the movements, thereby further strengthening the upper back and the abdominal zone as well as greatly increasing your total body strength. You'll see that you will be working your arms in a different way, which increases resistance and helps to build bone mass. Also, over time the exercise will tone the lower body and smooth down "saddlebags" (the fat that women typically store along the sides of their upper thighs and buttocks).

GLIDING BUTTERFLY

START   Lie on your stomach with your forehead resting on the mat. Extend your arms in front of you on the mat, palms facing down. [**1**

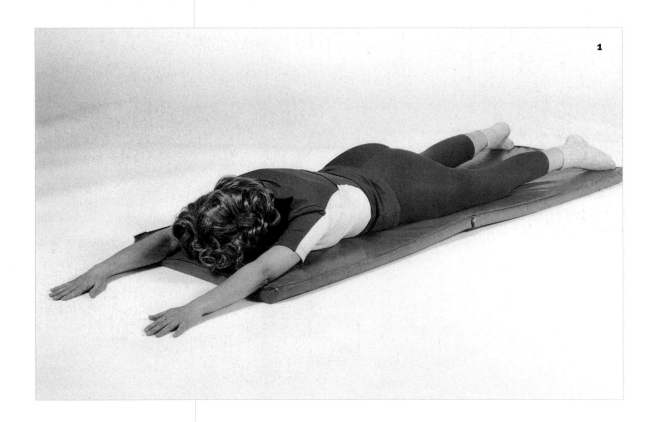

1

gliding butterfly/
heel beats combo

THE MOVEMENT

- Push your pubic bone into the mat by contracting your abdominal muscles, pulling them back toward your spine.

- With your arms extended in front of you, pull your shoulders back, elongate your neck, then lift your arms and slowly raise your chest off the mat. [2

- Keep the back of your neck elongated, chin slightly tucked in, with eyes focused downward.

- Bend and retract your elbows, palms facing down, as you pinch your shoulder blades together and down. [3

- Hold as you count out loud for three seconds.

- Glide your arms out again as you count out loud for three seconds. [4

- Repeat three times.

- Return to the starting position and then perform Heel Beats (following).

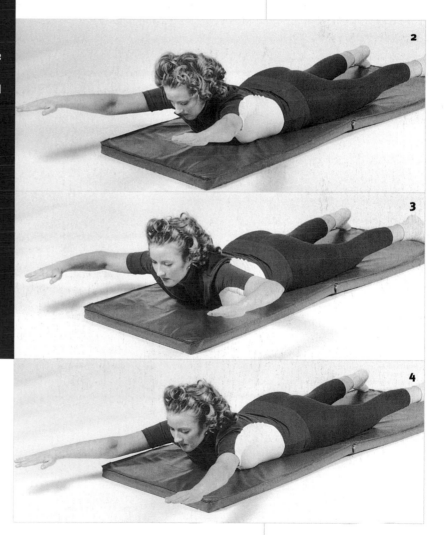

HEEL BEATS

START   Lie on your stomach with the backs of your hands creating a pillow for your forehead and press your pubic bone into the mat by recruiting your abdominal muscles. [**1**

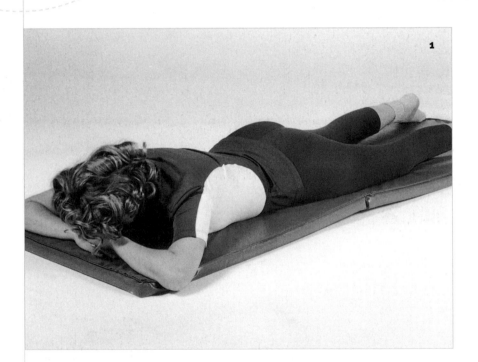

THE MOVEMENT

- Lift your legs, a little wider than shoulder-width apart, off the mat to buttock level. [2
- Click your heels together quickly, then back to shoulder-width apart, with toes turned outward. Repeat this in-out motion as many times as you can as you count out loud to thirty. [3
- Return your legs to the mat and repeat the Gliding Butterfly.

  Perform another thirty-count Heel Beats and finish with a Gliding Butterfly. You'll be doing a total of three Gliding Butterflies and two Heel Beats.

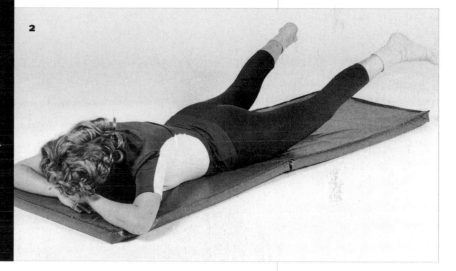

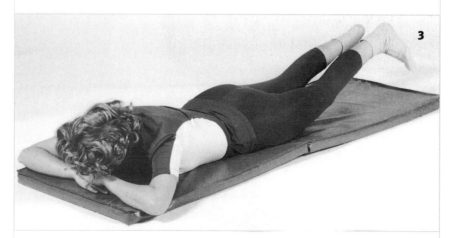

TIP:

- If you feel any discomfort in your lower back, push your pubic bone further into the mat, which will tighten the abdominals and provide more stability.

exercise **six**

THE PURPOSE   A stable spine, supple hips and a strong torso equal a long, elegant stride. This very effective series of exercises from the Core Foundation delivers even more impact because it uses ankle weights. The addition of weight to the Foot Circles strengthens the hip abductor muscles, which hold the hip in the proper alignment. Good alignment ensures that the cartilage, the cushiony substance that protects your joints, doesn't shift out of position, which helps protect you from osteoarthritis. It also guarantees that the hips bear weight evenly when you walk, thereby prompting the creation of more bone cells and preventing osteoporosis.

In a short while, you will find that this trio is giving you some cosmetic benefits, too—toning your outer thighs and buttocks and minimizing any saddlebags you may have.

Begin with one-pound weights for a week or two and then try two pounds.

PART ONE: HAMSTRING SIDE KICK

START   Put an ankle weight on your right leg. Lie on your left side, propped on the left elbow. Raise your upper body, contract your abdominal muscles, and support your weight on the left forearm, which is flat on the mat. Keep your left fist on the mat as well. Your legs should be straight, one on top of the other, at a 45 degree angle from your torso.

Place your right palm on the mat in front of you, your right forearm against your tightened abdomen, with the elbow pressed against the pelvic bone to prevent the tendency to roll backward. [1

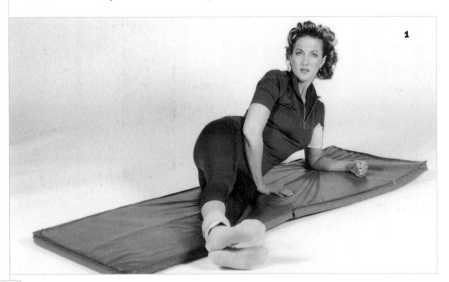

1

three-part weighted
pelvic stabilizer

THE MOVEMENT

- Lift your right leg six inches. [2
- Gently kick forward as far as possible with foot flexed, maintaining contact of the right elbow with the pelvis. [3
- Return to the starting position.
- Repeat six times as you count out loud to six.

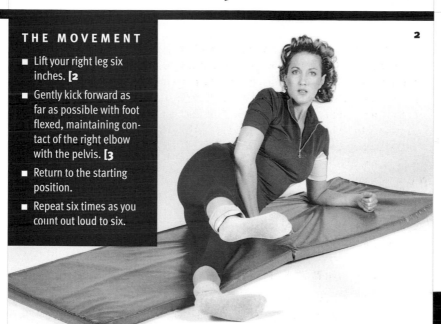

2

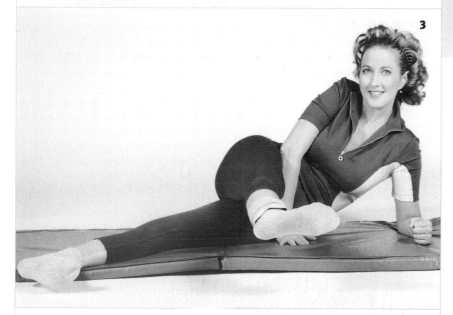

3

Make Sure You Don't:

- Slump forward.
- Roll back.

exercise **six**

PART TWO: GLUTEAL TONER

START Lying on your left side in the starting position, flex your right foot and lift your right leg six inches. **[1**

THE MOVEMENT

- Kick your leg backward. **[2**
- Return to the starting position.
- Repeat six times as you count out loud to six.

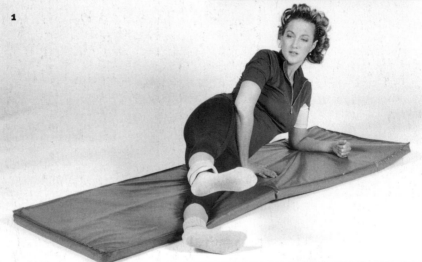

Make Sure You Don't:

Arch your back by kicking your leg too far behind you.

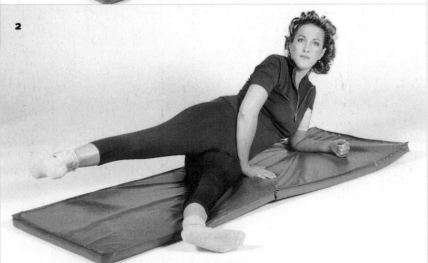

three-part weighted pelvic stabilizer

PART THREE: FOOT CIRCLES

START Lying on your left side in the starting position, rotate your right leg so the toes are flexed up toward the ceiling. [1

THE MOVEMENT

- Lift your right leg six inches, maintaining contact of the right elbow with the pelvis.
- Circle your leg clockwise, clicking your right heel against your left foot six times as you count out loud to six. Then circle counterclockwise six times as you count out loud to six.
- Repeat all three exercises on the opposite leg.

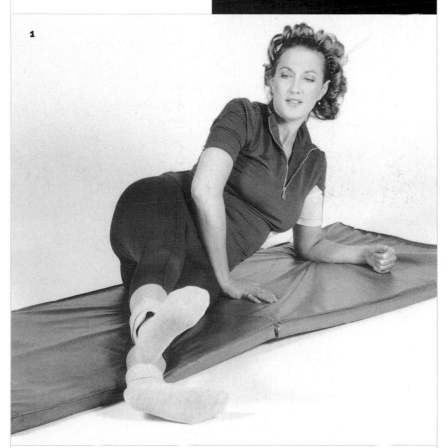

1

FORM CHECK:

- To maintain proper alignment, be sure your top forearm is braced against your pelvis the entire time.

TIPS:

- If you're unable to lift your leg to the proper height, lift it as high as you're able.
- If you can't continue for the allotted number of repetitions, take a brief rest and then continue.
- If you still have difficulty, reduce the size of the ankle weights.

NOTE: *Remove your ankle weights for the next exercise.*

exercise **seven**

FORM CHECK:

- Keep your shoulders down on the mat and your chin tucked in, which helps elongate your neck.

- Between each repetition of the stretch, be sure to release your knee a bit. This reduces the muscle tension, allowing the hamstring a chance to stretch further each time.

THE PURPOSE   I always give the hamstrings a lot of attention because these large muscles need it. Repeating this exercise from the Core Foundation will give you greater range of motion and will help protect you from lower-back discomfort.

Remember: All four parts of the exercise are performed on the one side before switching to the other.

PART ONE: KNEE TO CHEST STRETCH

START   Lie on your back with your knees bent and feet flat on the mat. Arms are by your sides, palms down. **[1**

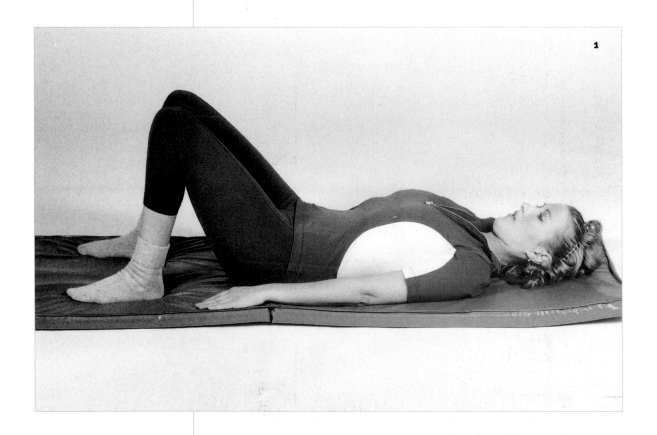

1

four-part progressive hamstring stretch

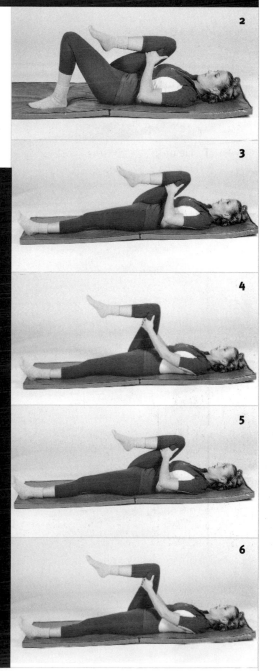

2

3

4

5

6

TIP:

- Take your thigh back as far as you can while still keeping your back flat on the floor. You may feel some discomfort but it will disappear as you become more flexible.

THE MOVEMENT

- Contract your abdominal muscles, elongate the back of your neck and press your lower back into the mat. *You will maintain this contraction and elongation through all four parts of the exercise.*

- Wrap your hands behind your right thigh and gently pull the right knee toward your chest. [2

- Hold the position as you count out loud to six and then release it.

- Slowly slide your left leg down along the mat. [3

- Release your right thigh to a 90 degree angle. [4

- Then gently pull the right thigh back to your chest. Hold the position as you count out loud to six and then release it. [5

- Repeat the stretch three times while your left leg remains flat on the mat. End by releasing the right thigh to a 90 degree angle in preparation for the next exercise. [6

PART TWO: STRAIGHT-LEG PRESSURE-ON, PRESSURE-OFF HAMSTRING STRETCH

FORM CHECK:

■ Be sure your shoulders are kept on the mat.

■ Keep your abdominal muscles tightened so that your lower back remains in contact with the mat at all times. If you feel strain in your back, bending the working leg slightly will help.

THE MOVEMENT

■ Straighten your right leg up as far as you can with both hands behind the knee while the left leg remains flat on the floor. [1

■ Bend your knee so your shin drops to a horizontal position and then return the leg to the vertical position. Repeat this motion six times as you count out loud to six. [2

■ End with your leg straight up in preparation for the next exercise. [3

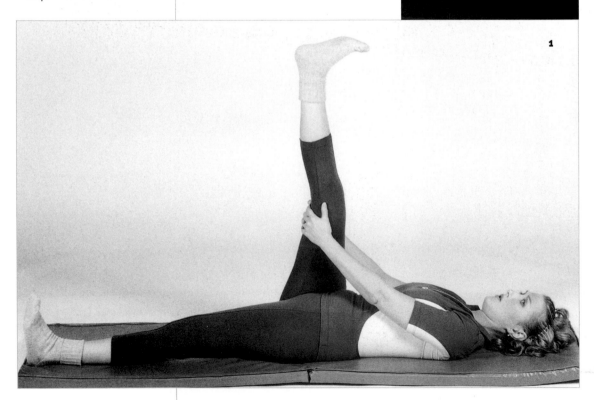

1

four-part progressive hamstring stretch

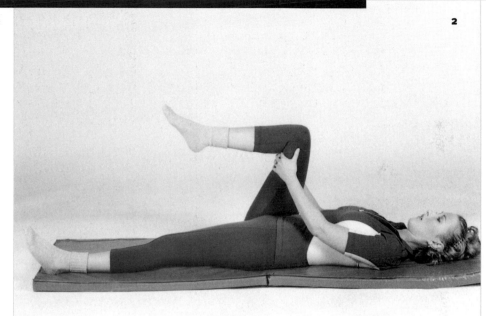

2

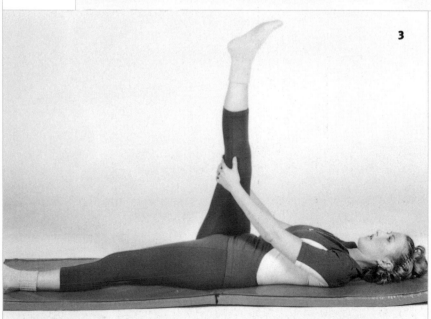

3

exercise **seven**
CONT.

PART THREE:
ANKLE PUMP

THE MOVEMENT

- Flex and release your foot as you count out loud to six. [**1**
- Finish with your leg straight up and foot flexed, which will take you into the next exercise. [**2**

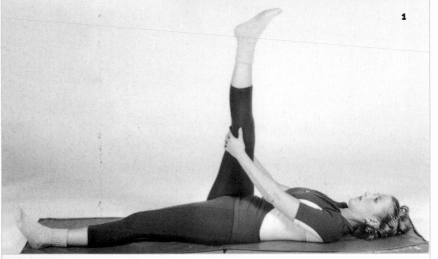

1

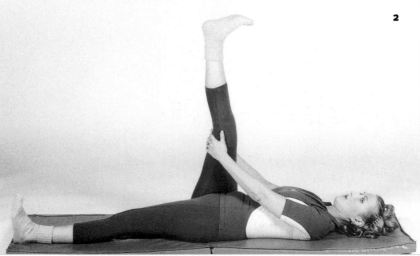

2

FORM CHECK:

- Be sure to contract your abdominals as you perform the exercise so that your lower back presses into the mat.
- Keep your shoulders on the mat to help maintain proper alignment. Place a pillow under your head if you cannot keep your shoulders down otherwise.

TIP:

- You may feel some discomfort behind your knee or in your hamstring as you perform the exercise. This will disappear as you gradually become more flexible.

four-part progressive hamstring stretch

THE MOVEMENT

- Lower your arms and brace them by your sides, palms down. [1
- Press your back into the mat, maximally tighten your buttocks and left thigh and keep your foot flexed. Hold the position as you count out loud to six.
- Keeping the contraction in all your muscles, slowly lower your leg, as you count out loud to six, until it comes to rest on the mat. [2 [3
- Repeat all four exercises with your other leg.

PART FOUR:
STEEL THIGHS

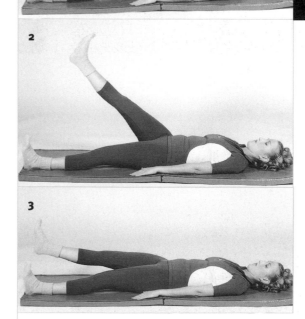

TIP:

- Make sure to keep your back pressed into the mat, especially when lowering the leg.
- If you can't keep your back pressed into the mat, place both hands under your buttocks for support.

exercise **eight**

THE PURPOSE This isometric position strengthens and tones the upper and lower abdominal muscles as it stretches lower back muscles, tones pelvic floor muscles and elongates the hamstrings—all without straining your neck. It will, however, tone the back and front muscles of the neck.

Note: The breathing directions are slightly different from what you have been doing in other exercises.

START Lie on your back with your legs in the air at a 90 degree angle, knees bent slightly. Keep your heels touching and your toes facing slightly outward. Keep your arms straight at your sides on the mat, palms up. Contract your abdominal muscles, elongate the back of your neck and press your lower back into the mat. **[1**

FORM CHECK:

- Be sure to keep your legs at a 90 degree angle and not angled out in front of you. If you lower them, the strong gravitational pull may prevent you from holding the proper position and can strain your lower back.

- If the exercise is too difficult, bring your legs closer to your trunk to lessen the resistance.

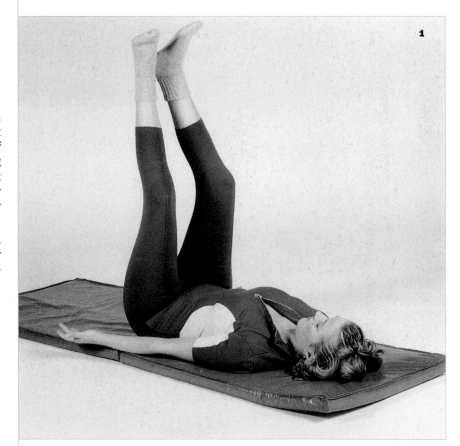

1

the mermaid

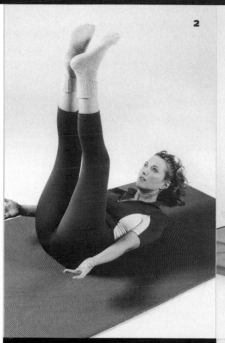

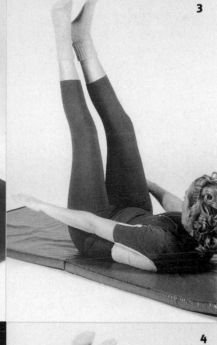

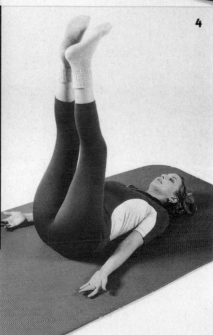

THE MOVEMENT

- Lift your head, shoulders and upper back off the mat as high as you can go. Raise your arms to the height of your hips. [2
- Pulse your arms, palms up, for the count of six, breathing in, and then palms down, breathing out, for the count of six. [3
- Repeat six times.
- Leaving your legs in the starting position, lower your upper body to the mat. [4

exercise **nine**

THE PURPOSE   Both this exercise, and the Lying Spinal Twist that follows, are included after the Mermaid to stretch out back muscles that you have just worked. This will prevent back spasms and free any compressed joints, disks, nerves or muscles.

START   Lie on your back with knees bent, feet flat on the mat, with the palms of your hands resting on your thighs. Elongate your neck, tuck your chin and make sure your shoulders are on the mat. Keep your abdominal muscles tightened and your lower back pressed down. [1

FORM CHECK:

- Shoulders should remain on the mat the entire time.
- Don't rock and roll your spine.

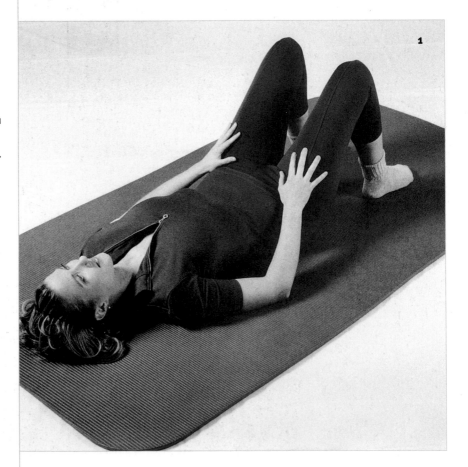

double knees to chest

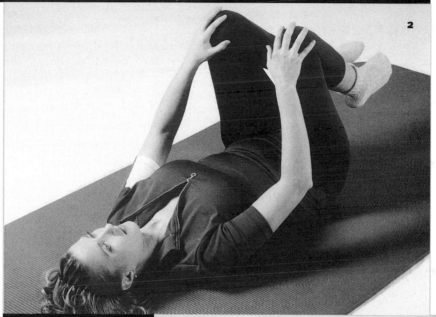

2

TIP:

- Be sure to breathe deeply. This will make it easier to bring your knees closer to your chest.

THE MOVEMENT

- Slowly pull your knees toward your chest. [2
- Hold the position as you count out loud to six and then release them to the starting position. [3
- Repeat three times.

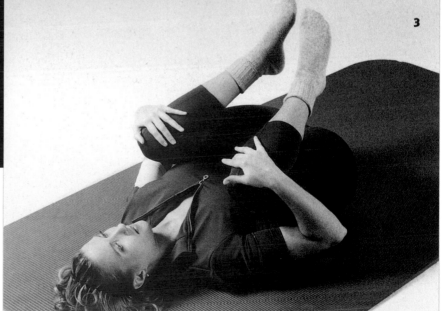

3

exercise **ten**

THE PURPOSE   This exercise will help stop any feeling of achiness resulting from the workout you gave your back muscles in preceding exercises, particularly the Mermaid.

START   Lie on your back with your face looking up at the ceiling. Bent knees are together, ankles are touching and feet are flat on the mat. Keep your arms straight out to the sides at shoulder height, so your body forms the letter T. Elongate your neck and make sure your shoulders are on the mat. Contract your abdominal muscles and press your lower back into the mat. **[1**

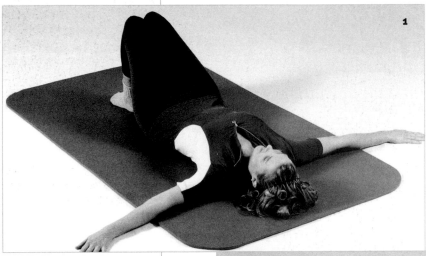

FORM CHECK:

- Be sure to keep your shoulders on the mat.

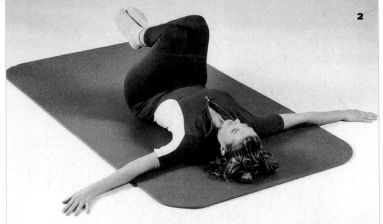

lying spinal twist

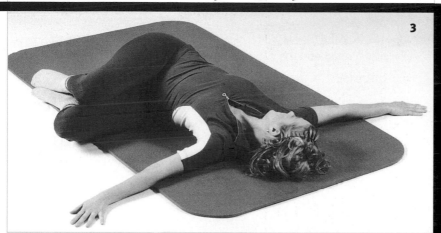

3

THE MOVEMENT

- Gradually lift the knees to your chest. **[2**
- Slowly drop both legs to the left side and rotate your head to the right side, keeping both shoulders flat on the mat. **[3**
- Hold the position as you count out loud to six and then pull your knees back to your chest. **[4**
- Repeat on the opposite side. **[5**
- Perform a total of four twists, two for each side.

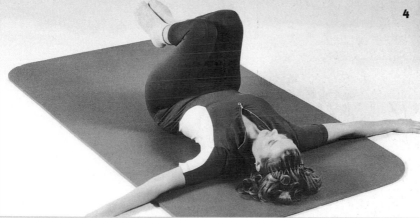

4

TIP:

- As you gain flexibility, both sides of your body will feel equally relaxed.

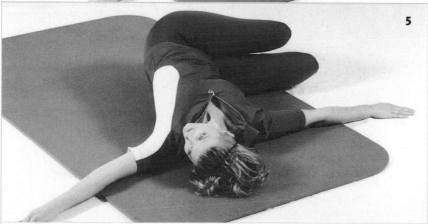

5

exercise **eleven**

When you breathe deeply, you automatically function better. Your lungs fill with oxygen, which is carried through the bloodstream to every cell. Deep breathing also alleviates muscular tension you may not even be aware of, especially during a stressful day.

Do it exactly as you did in Exercise #3.

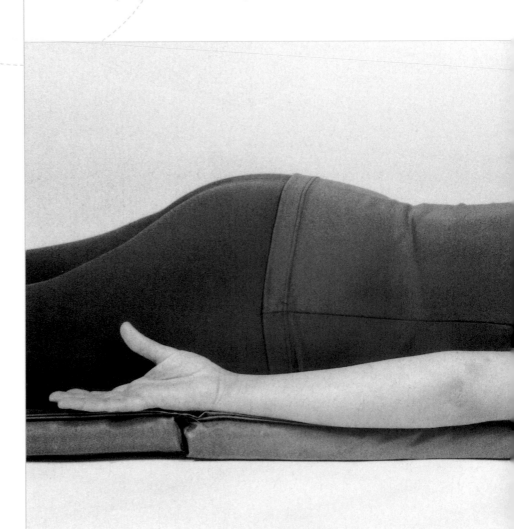

belly breath

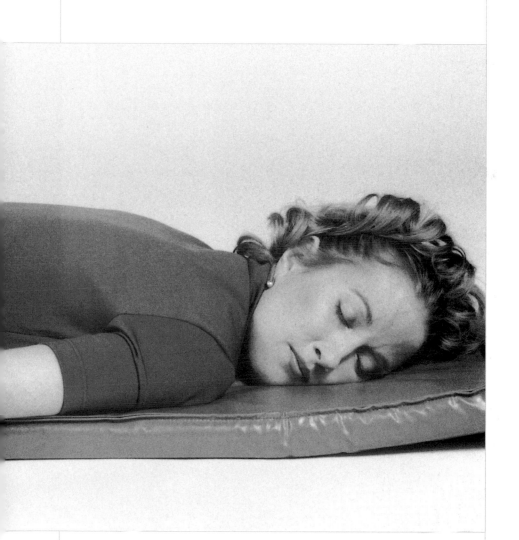

exercise **twelve**

THE PURPOSE This exercise will provide better alignment when you sit and stand. You've probably done these coordinated arm and leg swimming motions in the water. Doing them on land, where your body is working against gravity, will cool the hot spot muscles in the neck, shoulders and upper back and lower back while it works the muscles of the buttocks, thighs and calves. Being a "swimmer" will give you more powerful shoulders and legs along with better defined abdominal muscles.

It may take some time to develop the arm/leg coordination but the results are really worth the effort.

START Lie on your stomach with your forehead resting on the backs of your hands. Tighten your abdominals and press your pubic bone into the mat. **[1**

FORM CHECK:

■ Be sure to keep your pubic bone pressed into the mat by tightening your abdominals. This will keep you from rocking from side to side.

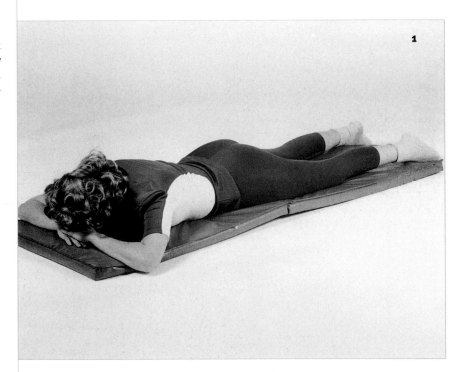

1

the swimmer

THE MOVEMENT

Lower body only

- Lift one leg up at a time, with straight knees, from the mat to the height of your buttocks. [2

- Then lift both legs, keeping them slightly elevated. Alternate moving your legs up and down in a flutter kick. Do as many as you can as you count out loud to thirty. [3

- Return to the starting position. [4

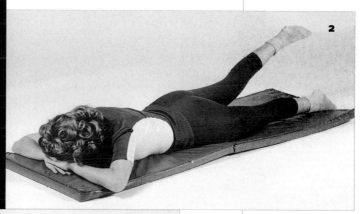

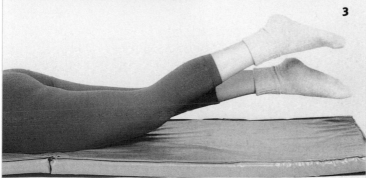

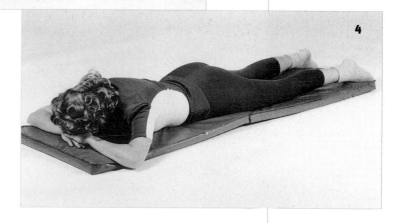

THE MOVEMENT

Upper body only

- Extend your arms out in front of you, palms down. Push your pubic bone into the mat.

- Lift your arms several inches and raise your head and chest off the mat as far as you comfortably can with your face looking straight ahead, chin slightly tucked so that you don't compress the muscles at the back of your neck. **[1**

- Start the breaststroke, sweeping your arms out to the sides with elbows bent and moving them as far back as possible, then return them to the starting position. **[2**

- Continue the breaststroke motion, doing as many as you can as you count out loud to thirty.

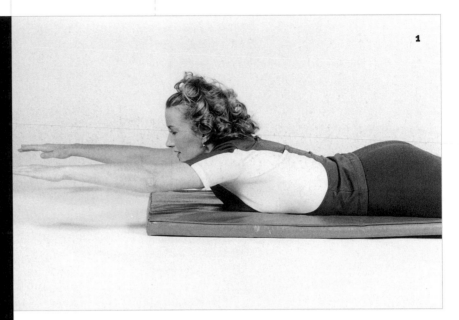

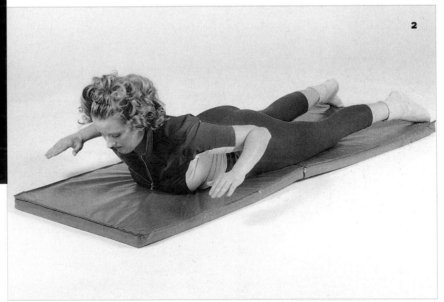

the swimmer

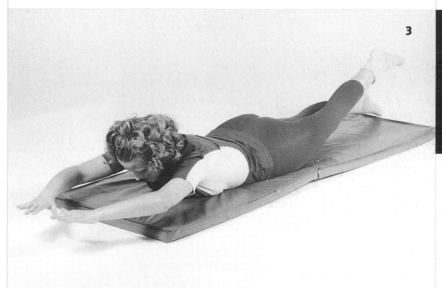

3

THE MOVEMENT

Upper and lower body

- Combine the flutter kicking and breaststroke motions. Do as many as you can as you count out loud to thirty. [3 [4

TIP:

- If you can't do the prescribed number of strokes, just work your way up gradually.

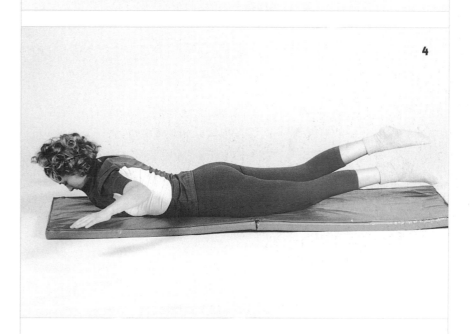

4

exercise **thirteen**

FORM CHECK:

- As you begin your stretch, imagine your spine as a banana that you are slowly peeling from your neck, mid-back, then lower back.

- Instead of tightening your buttocks as you lift off the mat, which limits the spinal extension, just press up with your arms into the range that is most comfortable. With each repetition, attempt to press up higher, keeping your buttocks relaxed.

- Keep your back relaxed and "flaccid." Don't hunch your shoulders together. Let your arms do the work.

- Try not to scrunch the muscles at the back of your neck together as you look up at the ceiling. Think about elongating the back of the neck at the same time that you are tilting it back, and pushing up and out from the chest.

As you know by now, this effective stretch not only loosens up your lower back—it feels *so* good.

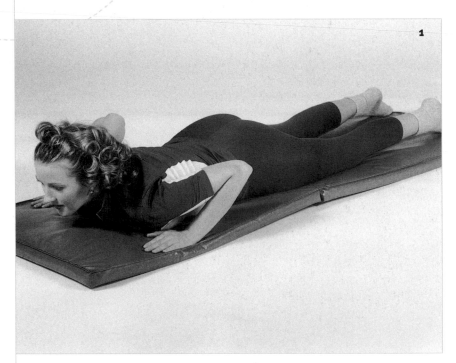

THE MOVEMENT

- Push up, tilting your head back slightly, in the sequence of forehead, nose and chin. [1

- Face forward as you rise, pushing up on your arms and opening your chest, keeping your pubic bone pushed into the mat while relaxing the buttocks as best you can. [2

- Slowly arch your spine backward, straightening, but not locking, your elbows.

- Roll your head back until you are looking straight up at the ceiling. [3

- Hold the position as you count out loud to three and then descend slowly to the mat. [4

- Repeat six times.

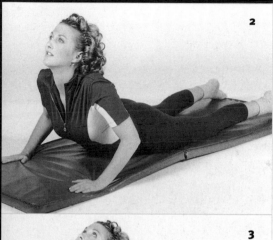

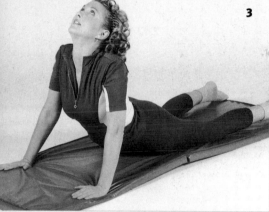

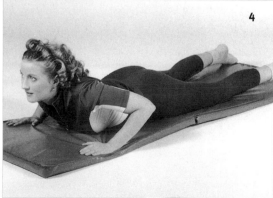

exercise **fourteen**

THE PURPOSE   The following facial muscle exercises will tone and strengthen most of the muscles of the face and neck. The more you perform each facial exercise, the closer you will come to achieving—and maintaining—a firm, smooth face. The exercises tone the muscles of the cheekbones and neck, shrink jowls and help minimize folds between the nose and mouth. And they help to relax the horizontal furrows in the forehead and reduce the vertical crease between eyebrows.

The trio also helps relieve the pain and discomfort of frontal headaches, facial tension and jaw discomfort including nocturnal grinding. It's also a great tension reliever if speaking in public makes you clench facial muscles.

Remember: It takes seventeen muscles to smile and forty-three muscles to frown. Happiness and joy of life are still two of the best ways to improve facial beauty.

START   Do the following exercises while sitting cross-legged on the mat, with your hands resting in your lap.

tongue stretch

THE MOVEMENT

- Stick out your tongue, keeping it down and extended over the lower lip, as far as possible. At the same time, without moving your head, gaze up, trying to see as far as you can behind your head.

- Silently count to six and then release.

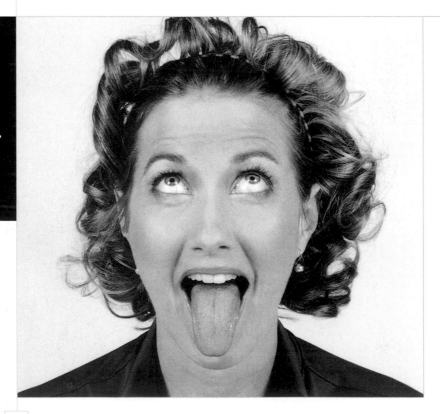

about-face: tongue stretch, x's and o's, line eraser

THE MOVEMENT

- Say "X" in the most exaggerated way you can, causing the jaw to protrude. [1
- Hold as you count to three to yourself and then release.
- Say "O" in the most exaggerated way and, holding the position, then try to smile. [2, [3
- Hold as you count to three to yourself and then release.
- Alternate "X" and "O," repeating each three times.

X's and O's

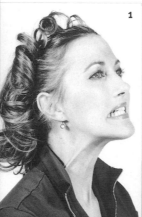

1

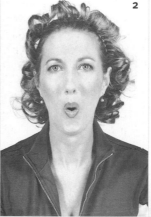

2

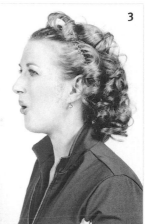

3

FORM CHECK:

- Perform a test run of *X's* and *O's*, as well as the following Line Eraser, while looking in the mirror.

line eraser

1

2

THE MOVEMENT

- Close your eyes.
- Gently put your index and middle fingers just below your eyebrows. [1
- Press up gently on your eyebrows and scowl. [2
- Gently resist the pressure of your eyebrows against your fingers.
- Hold as you count out loud to six and then release.
- Repeat three times.

exercise **fifteen**

After your rigorous workout, this exercise helps you relax all your muscles.
Do it exactly as you did before.

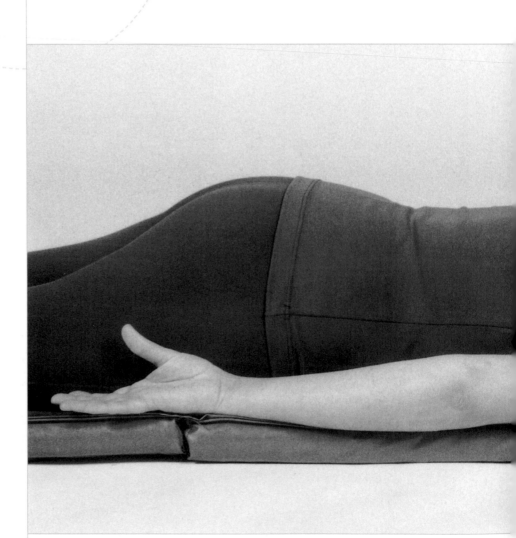

belly breath finale

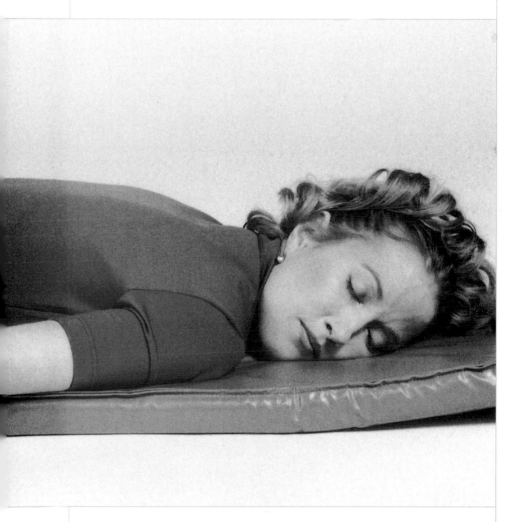

GOOD FOR YOU!

You're stronger and straighter than ever before, and you are looking—and feeling—younger.

the intermediate core

1. Head-to-Toe Prep

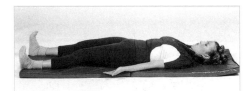

2. Dead Bugs

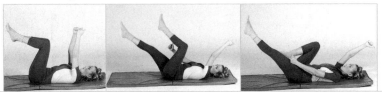

3. Belly Breath

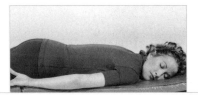

4. The Cobra

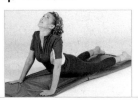

5. Gliding Butterfly/Heel Beats Combo

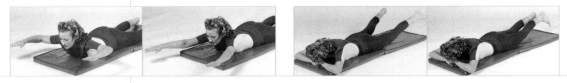

6. Three-Part Weighted Pelvic Stabilizer

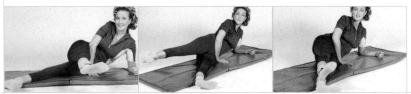

7. Four-Part Progressive Hamstring Stretch

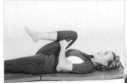 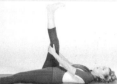 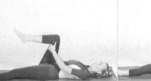 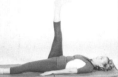 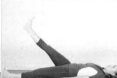

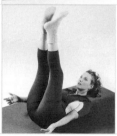

9. Double Knees to Chest

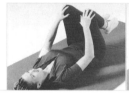 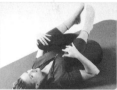

8. The Mermaid

10. Lying Spinal Twist

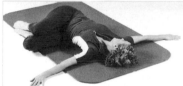 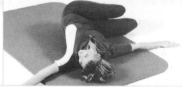 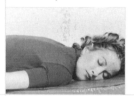

11. Belly Breath

12. The Swimmer

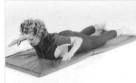 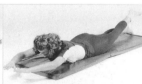 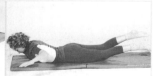

13. The Cobra **14.** About-Face

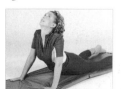 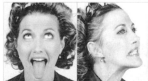

15. Belly Breath Finale

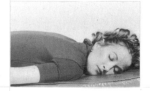

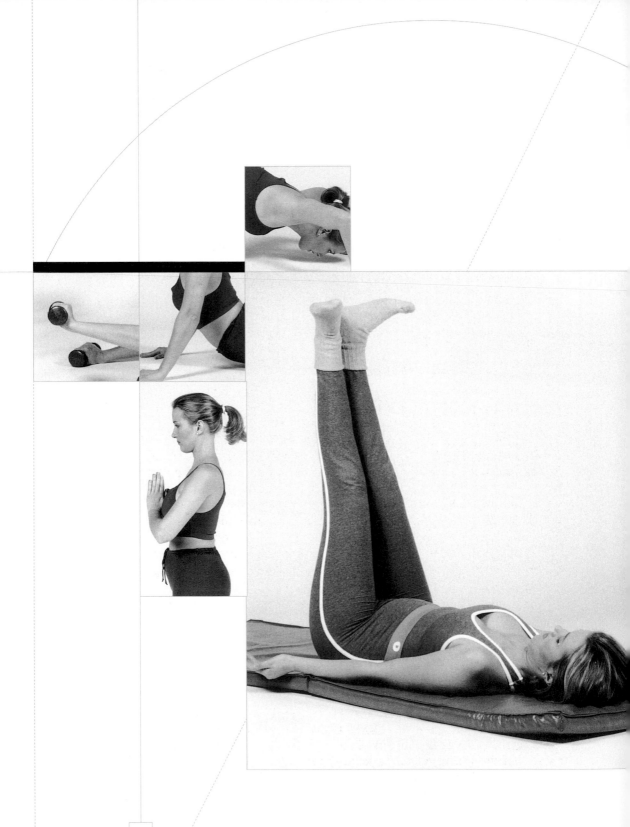

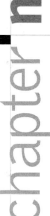

The Ultimate Core

After doing the Intermediate Core for at least three weeks, you may be ready to try the Ultimate Core. The most demanding of the three programs, this set of exercises packs more strenuous motions into fewer exercises. Many of my patients reach this level. More than a few are past sixty; some are in their eighties.

Now that your back and abdominal muscles have repeatedly performed isometric strengthening throughout the previous Core Programs, you are ready for something new. By adding dumbbells to your workout, and using heavier ankle weights, you will give your extremities more of an isotonic workout. At the same time, you will continue strengthening your torso with even more intense isometric contractions. The combination will further enhance your ability to move throughout the day with ease and grace, and you will have an increasingly well-toned body coupled with amazing strength and vitality.

The Ultimate Core includes three new exercises. More challenging variations of five exercises you are already familiar with are also here.

Remember: Unless otherwise stated, the exercises that are done while lying on your back are performed with your chin retracted, your abdominal muscles hollowed out and your pelvis slightly tilted.

Before you begin, place your ankle weights and dumbbells near the mat, so that they will be ready for you when you need them. Depending on how strong you are, you will be using two- to five-pound dumbbells and two- to five-pound ankle weights. Start low and build up to the higher weights as you build your strength in the weeks to come.

the **ultimate** core

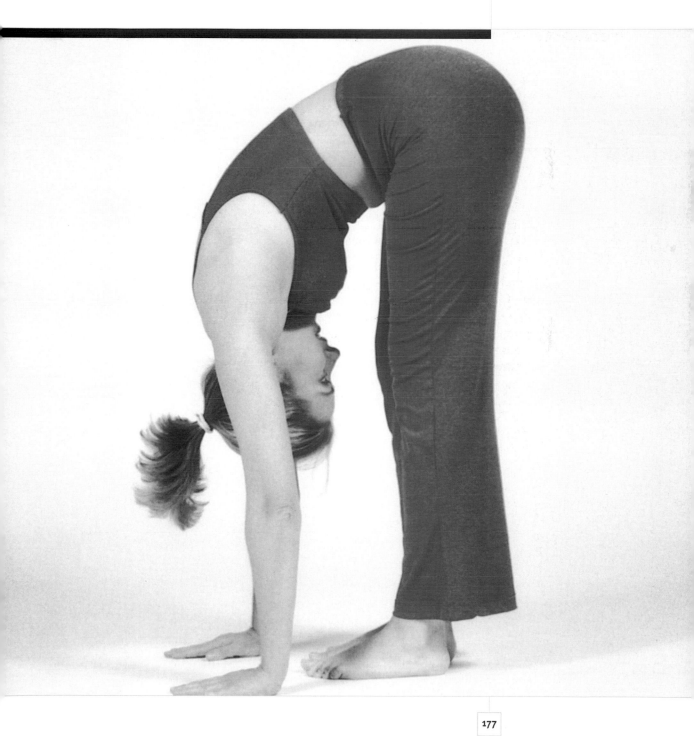

exercise **one**

THE PURPOSE   Both of the previous Core Programs prepared you, by improving your muscle flexibility, for this classic yoga exercise. The Sun Salutation, which literally means "to bow to the sun" in Sanskrit, is a sequence of fourteen separate, flowing movements that will have you alternately bending and stretching forward and backward. Elongating everything that tends to shorten and strengthening everything that tends to weaken, it makes you both supple and strong.

This phenomenal set of movements creates the perfect balance between extension and flexion throughout the major joints, making sure that they are aligned. By ensuring correct weight bearing in the spine, hips and wrists, this wonderful exercise also helps prevent osteoarthritis and osteoporosis. The stretches are so encompassing that even the bottoms of your feet are included!

These gentle body movements enhance circulation of blood and lymph, and expand your respiratory capacity. They also increase joint lubrication and spinal suppleness, and improve overall balance and coordination.

For lifelong flexibility, this dynamic head-to-toe stretching routine is the one that I recommend you do every day. It has eliminated, or significantly reduced, the morning stiffness that most of my patients complain about. And it only takes two minutes a day to perform—a small investment for a great return.

Even if you find the rest of the Ultimate Core a bit too demanding, please do the Sun Salutation and then go back and do the exercises of the Intermediate Core without the Head-to-Toe Prep.

One last note: The breathing sequence for the Sun Salutation is different from that of the other exercises, so read the instructions a couple of times before you begin.

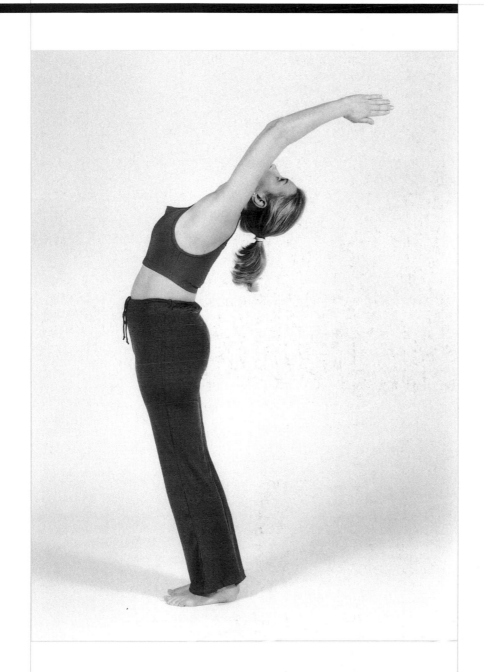

THE MOVEMENT

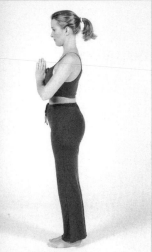
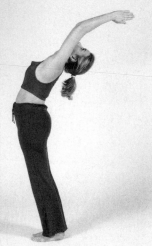
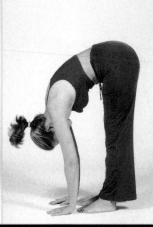

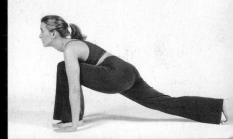

1. Mountain. Begin by standing, feet together, pressing down into the floor with your weight evenly divided between the balls and heels of your feet, and your hands in front of your chest in prayer position.

2. Arms Up. Take a deep breath, 1–2–3, and as you inhale, raise your arms up overhead in one motion, keeping the palms of your hands together. Lift and expand your chest as you gently arch your head and back as far as you comfortably can while exhaling.

3. Head-to-Knees. Bend forward at the waist, dropping your head toward your knees, stretching your arms and bringing your hands to the tops of your feet (or on the mat alongside your feet, depending on your flexibility). Bend your knees if necessary. Hold this position as you take a deep breath in and out.

4. Lunge. Move your right leg back into a lunge, keeping the right knee slightly bent and your left knee directly above your left ankle. Lengthen your body upward, looking up and lifting your chin.

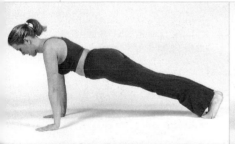

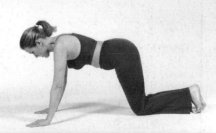

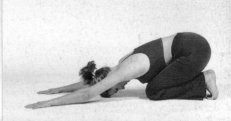

5. Plank.
As you inhale, move your left foot back to join the right and straighten both legs so you are now in the classic push-up position. Your abdomen should be tightly contracted, your spine in a straight line, neither arched nor rounded. Hold the position and exhale, contracting the abdomen even more.

6. Table.
Inhale and drop your knees to the mat.

7. Child's Pose.
Sit back on your heels with your arms outstretched, and your toes tucked under you to stretch the bottoms of your feet.

Continue ··· ❯

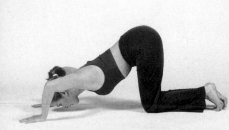 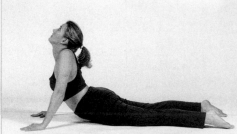 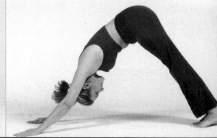

8. The Cat.
With your hands in the same outstretched position, skim your nose along the mat and arch your back like a cat as you exhale and glide forward.

9. The Cobra.
As your chest reaches the mat, uncurl your toes so that the tops of your feet lie flat on the mat. Inhale as you slowly lift your head back. Push up by extending your arms, bending backward at the waist to arch your back. Your buttocks remain relaxed and the pelvis firmly on the mat if possible. Bend back as far as it feels comfortable, as you straighten—not lock—your arms. Exhale.

10. Downward Dog (Inverted V).
Inhale, and use your arms, hips and feet to lift your tailbone so that you are bent over in an inverted V position. Straighten your arms and legs and press your hands and feet firmly into the mat, lengthening from your shoulders to your hands, and your tailbone to your feet. Your heels should reach back as far as they can toward the mat.

Hold this stretch for another deep inhale and exhale.

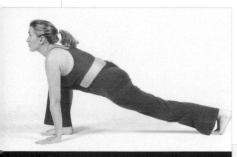

FORM CHECK:

- Exhale as you bend backward or whenever exerting yourself.
- Tighten your buttocks to stabilize and protect your spine.
- The postures should flow smoothly from one position to the next.

11. Lunge.

On your next inhalation, bend your right knee and step forward until the right foot is parallel to the palms of your hands. If you can't get it all the way there, pick it up and move it forward until it's even with your hands. The right knee should be directly above the right ankle. Your left leg should be stretched back, with your knee slightly bent and your toes tucked under in a push-off position.

Exhale and drop your hips slightly to further lengthen your body and stretch the front of your upper thigh.

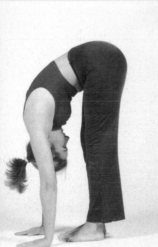

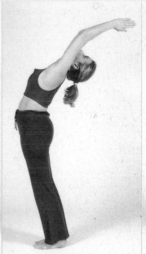

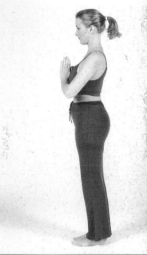

12. Head-to-Knees.

Inhale and bring your left foot forward to meet your right and straighten both legs as your palms remain flat on the mat and your head drops to your knees.

Exhale. If you can't get your palms to the mat, bend your knees until you can.

13. Hands Up.

Inhale, bend your knees slightly, squeeze your buttocks together and allow your arms to hang loosely, palms together, as you roll up, one vertebra at a time.

14. Arching.

Bringing your arms overhead with your hands close together, tilt your head back and allow your chest to rise and expand as you exhale.

15. Mountain.

Keeping your palms together, bend your elbows and lower your hands to your chest, bringing them back to prayer position.

Inhale for four seconds.

Hold for the count of seven.

Exhale for the count of eight.

Repeat the entire sequence, this time starting with your left leg.

exercise **two**

THE PURPOSE   Doing this exercise will give you greater ease, grace and strength as you move from a sitting to a standing position or go up and down stairs. The extra leg power will be useful if you're active in any sports, too. And it will also help you with lifting. (As a mother of two children I can attest that this really works.) In addition to developing the muscles of your hips, thighs and calves, squats target the abdominal zone and lower back.
Note: Have your three-pound hand weights ready.

FORM CHECK:

- Keep your feet flat on the mat and drop your body weight behind your knees to prevent straining your knees.

- Sit back as if you're hovering over a toilet seat.

- Women with tight heel cords: You will need to place a block of wood under your heels if your feet do not remain flat on the floor in the final position.

SQUEEZE PAIN AWAY:

- If you feel pain when you walk down stairs, try squeezing your buttocks as you descend. Doing this prevents your knees from rolling in toward each other, a position which strains the joints and gives you discomfort.

START Stand with your feet slightly wider than shoulder-width apart, abdominals contracted.

Hold a weight in each hand, with your palms facing in at your sides. **[1**

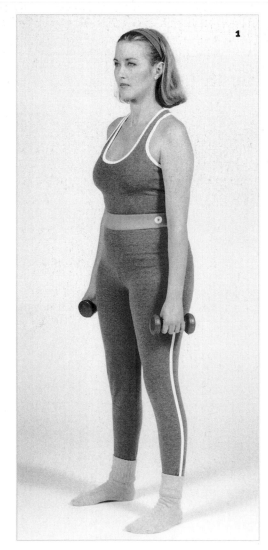

1

squats

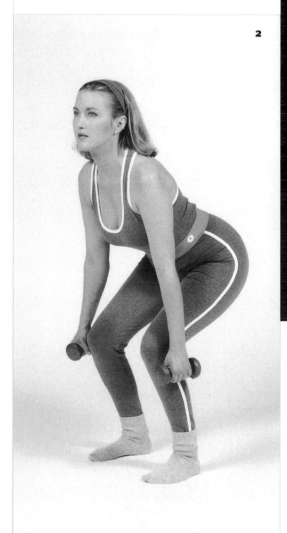

2

THE MOVEMENT

- Slowly bend your knees, keeping your feet flat on the mat, buttocks moving backward. Keep your kneecaps aligned over your second toes.

- Count out loud to three as you lower your body until your hands are near mid-calf level and your upper thighs are almost parallel to the mat. **[2**

- Pause momentarily.

- Push upward forcefully with your quadriceps as you count out loud to three. As you straighten to standing, lengthen your back and squeeze your buttocks, which isolates muscles of your hips, thighs and calves.

- Repeat eighteen times.

Note: Put your weights aside before going on to the next exercise.

Make Sure You Don't:

- Bend your knees past your toes. This will wear down the cartilage behind your knee-caps.

- Knock your knees together. This will strain the cartilage along the inside of joint surfaces of your knees.

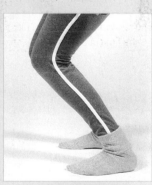

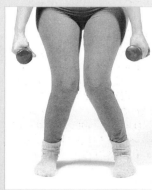

exercise **three**

FORM CHECK:

- Don't bend your elbows – keep them locked – when you bring them back behind your head.
- Be sure to keep your shoulders on the mat.
- If you feel that your torso is moving from side to side, it means that you are not keeping your abdominal muscles contracted.
- Press your back to the mat to maintain your stable position.
- Be sure to keep your thumbs pointed toward the ceiling – as if you were hitchhiking. This prevents damage to the rotator cuff muscles of your shoulders.

THE PURPOSE   An intensification of the Dead Bugs you performed in the Intermediate Core, this version takes abdominal strengthening up another notch. As you contract both your upper and lower abdominal muscles, you will be adding resistance by moving your arms and legs away from your core at the same time.

You may feel some initial discomfort but this will pass as your abdominal muscles adjust to the increased demands. Start by trying to do the exercise for a count of thirty and then work up to sixty.

START Lie on your back with your knees bent and your feet flat on the mat. Keep your arms bent with your palms on your abdomen. Keep the back of your neck elongated with the chin tucked down and the small of your back pressed into the mat. [1

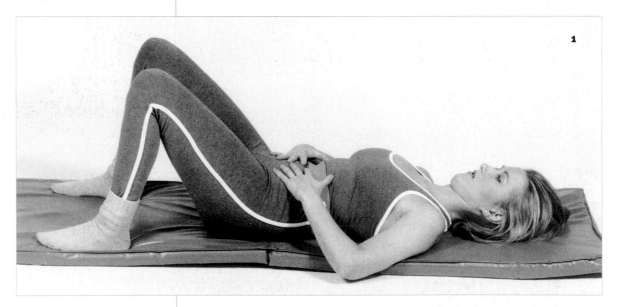

1

double dead bugs

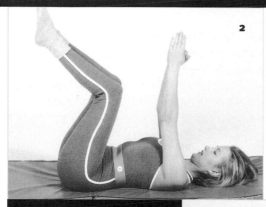

2

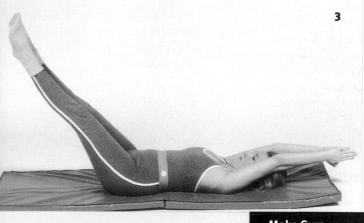

3

THE MOVEMENT PART ONE

- Contract your abdominal muscles.
- Lift your knees up toward your chest. Lift your arms straight up toward the ceiling, with your thumbs pointing up. **[2**

THE MOVEMENT PART TWO

- Contract your abdominal muscles. Move both legs out at a 45 degree angle while simultaneously lifting both arms back over and behind your head. **[3**
- Combine movements one and two, so that your arms and legs come together and apart like a clam opening and closing, being sure to keep your lower back pressed flat to the mat the whole time. Do as many as you can while counting out loud to thirty. Eventually you may work up to a count of sixty. **[4**

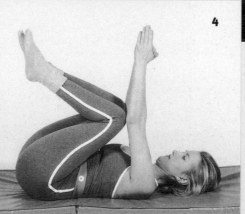

4

Make Sure You Don't:

- Arch your back.

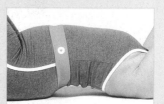

exercise **four**

Make Sure You Don't:

- Arch your back.
- Release the contraction in your abdominal muscles.

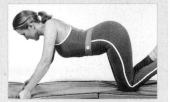

THE PURPOSE   Yes, these are the push-ups you tried and probably failed to do in school. But now you *can* do them because you have built up your upper body strength. (Boys could always do them because they started out with more upper body mass than you did). Push-ups do your body a lot of good. They help prevent osteoporosis throughout the upper extremities by ensuring correct weight bearing and bone building—particularly in the wrists. At the same time they tone and build up your arms.

Begin with the woman's push-up. When you can do eighteen repetitions move on to the classic version.

WOMAN'S PUSH-UP:

START   Kneel on the mat and cross your ankles. Extend your arms in front of you, fists or palms shoulder-width apart on the mat, and lower yourself into position. Tighten your abdomen, lengthen the back of your neck, and tuck your chin. [1

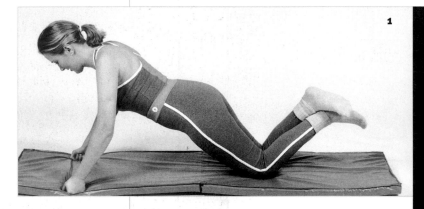

THE MOVEMENT

- Bend your elbows and lower your chest toward the mat, keeping your back, neck and head in a straight line. [2
- Hold the position briefly, then return slowly to the starting position.
- Count out loud on the push up as you repeat the movement six times. Gradually work your way up to eighteen reps, increasing six at a time.

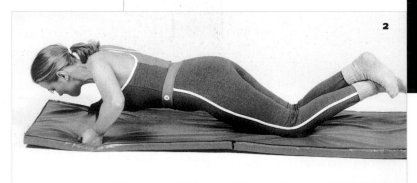

push-ups

CLASSIC PUSH-UP:

START   Place your fists or palms on the mat shoulder-width apart, and extend your legs straight out behind you, feet flexed so that your toes are tucked beneath you. Tighten your abdomen, lengthen the back of your neck and tuck your chin. [1

Make Sure You Don't:

- Arch your back.
- Hunch your back.

Either of these positions will strain your back.

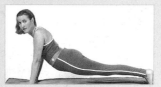

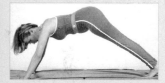

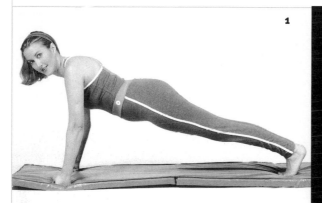

1

THE MOVEMENT

- Bend your elbows and lower your chest toward the mat keeping your back, neck and head in a straight line. Go as low as you can, but not so low that you allow your elbows to rise higher than your shoulders—which will be about four to six inches from the floor. [2

- Hold briefly, then return slowly to the starting position.

- Count out loud on the push up as you repeat the movement six times. Gradually work your way up to eighteen reps, increasing six at a time.

- Allow your wrists to rotate inward, toward your body. Doing so will strain your wrists.

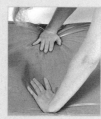

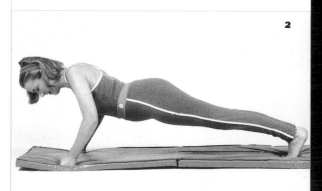

2

FORM CHECK:

- Tighten your abdominals and squeeze your buttocks to support your spine.
- Lower yourself only within the range that you can control.
- When you straighten your arms, don't lock your elbows.

exercise **five**

THE PURPOSE Adding hand weights, along with ankle weights, in this variation of the Core Foundation exercise promotes bone cell growth because of the additional force with which muscle pulls on bone. This two-part exercise also balances the hips and strengthens both the outer and inner thigh muscles as it tones the saddlebag and buttock areas. The result will be firmly sculpted thighs and taut buttocks.

Start with two-pound ankle weights and two-pound dumbbells. After three weeks, try three-pound ankle weights and three-pound dumbbells. After another three weeks, see if you can progress to five-pound weights and five-pound dumbbells.

BUTTERFLY WITH WEIGHTS

START Put on ankle weights and rest the dumbbells in your palms. Lie on your stomach with your forehead resting on the mat. Keep your arms at your sides, palms facing upward. **[1**

THE MOVEMENT

- Contract your abdominal muscles and push your pubic bone into the mat. Squeeze your shoulder blades together behind you. Keep the back of your neck elongated, chin slightly tucked in, with eyes focused downward.

- Slowly raise your chest off the mat as high as possible by pinching your shoulder blades together. At the same time, raise your arms to the level of your buttocks. **[2**

- Hold this position while counting out loud to six and release.

- Put down the dumbbells and perform Heel Beats (following).

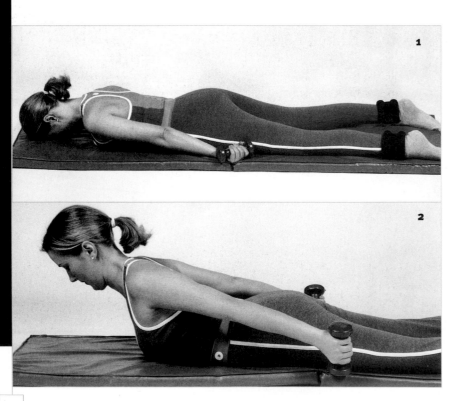

1

2

butterfly with weights/
heel beats with weights

HEEL BEATS WITH WEIGHTS

START   Lie on your stomach with the backs of your hands creating a pillow for your forehead and press your pubic bone into the mat by recruiting your abdominal muscles. [1

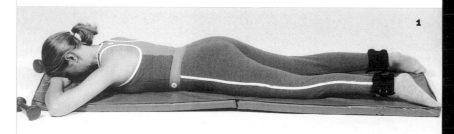

1

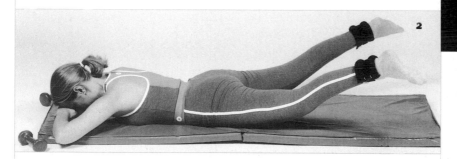

2

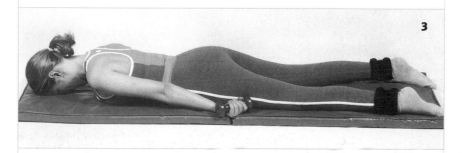

3

TIPS:

- If you feel any discomfort in your lower back, contract your stomach muscles to push your pubic bone farther into the mat.

- If discomfort continues, put a pillow under your stomach and push your pubic bone into the pillow.

  Note: Put your dumbbells aside in preparation for the next exercise. Choose ankle weights that are one or more pounds heavier than those you used in the Intermediate Core version of the Pelvic Stabilizer.

exercise **six**

THE PURPOSE   Using ankle weights that are heavier than the ones you used when you did this exercise before will further develop your legs and gluteal muscles. The musculature of your outer thighs and buttocks will become visible as saddlebags diminish even more.

Begin with three-pound ankle weights for each leg. Use them for three weeks and then increase the weights to four pounds per leg if you feel ready. Use the four-pound weights for three weeks and then try to increase to five pounds.

All three parts of the exercise are performed for the right side before switching to the left.

PART ONE: HAMSTRING SIDE KICK

START   Put on your ankle weights. Lie on your left side, propped on the left elbow. Raise your upper body, contract your abdominal muscles, and support your weight on the left forearm, which is flat on the mat. Keep your left fist flat on the mat as well. Keep your legs straight, one on top of the other, at a 45 degree angle from your torso.

Place your right palm on the mat in front you, your right forearm against your tightened abdomen, with the elbow pressed against the pelvic bone to eliminate the tendency to roll backward. **[1**

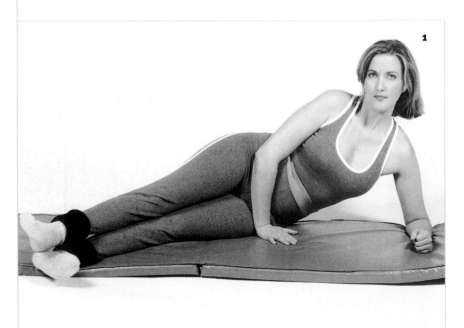

1

three-part advanced pelvic stabilizer

THE MOVEMENT

- Lift your right leg three inches and gently kick forward as far as possible with foot flexed, maintaining contact of the right elbow with the pelvis. [2
- Return to the starting position.
- Repeat six times as you count out loud to six.

FORM CHECK:

- It's important that you always keep a forearm braced against your pelvis. This constant contact ensures that you are in the right position to stretch your hamstrings, and it prevents you from overusing your hip flexors.

Make Sure You Don't:

- Slump forward.
- Roll back.

Doing either motion will prevent isolation of the muscles you want to work.

2

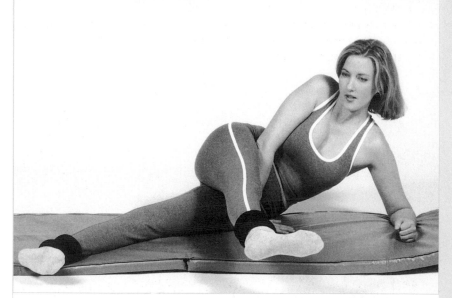

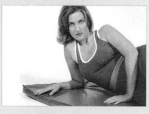

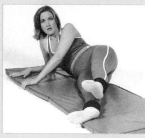

PART TWO:
GLUTEAL TONER

START Lying on your left side in the starting position, flex your foot and lift your right leg six inches. **[1**

THE MOVEMENT

- Kick your leg backward. **[2**
- Return to the starting position.
- Repeat six times as you count out loud to six.

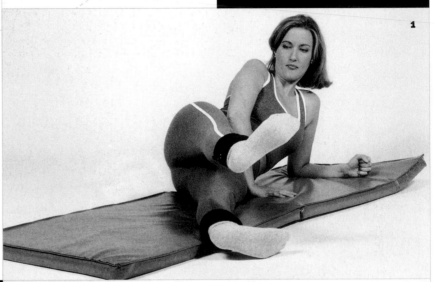

Make Sure You Don't:

Arch your back by extending your leg too far.

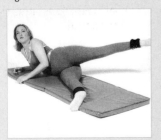

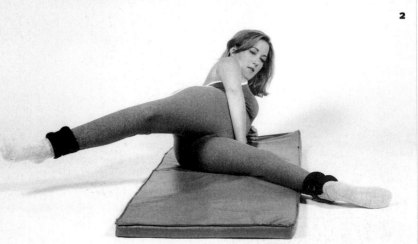

PART THREE: FOOT CIRCLES

START Lying on your left side in the starting position, rotate your right foot so your toes are flexed and pointing to the ceiling. **[1**

THE MOVEMENT

- Lift your leg six inches, maintaining contact between your right elbow and your pelvis. **[2**
- Circle your leg clockwise, clicking your right heel against your left foot six times as you count out loud to six. Then circle counterclockwise six times as you count out loud to six.
- Repeat all three exercises on the opposite leg.
  Note: Remove your ankle weights before going on to the next exercise.

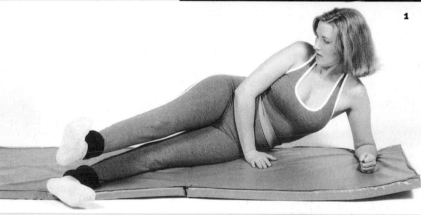

1

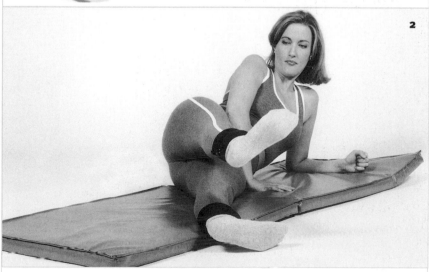

2

FORM CHECK:

- To maintain proper alignment, remember to keep your forearm positioned against your pelvis.

TIPS:

- If you're unable to lift your leg to the recommended height, just elevate it as high as you can.
- As you perform this exercise, the side of your buttock may become sore. Massage it for a few seconds after you've completed the exercise; it will feel better.
- If you can't continue for the allotted number of repetitions, take a brief rest and then continue.

exercise **seven**

THE PURPOSE What makes this different from the exercise in the Intermediate Core is the angle of your legs. Moving your legs farther from your torso, with straight knees, will greatly add to the intensity of the exercise. This will result in abdominal muscles that are stronger than ever and able to support you even better. This exercise is a terrific spine stabilizer, too.

Note: The directions for breathing are slightly different in this exercise.

START Lie on your back with your legs straight up in the air. Keep your heels touching, toes pointed outward and inner thighs pressed together as your legs form a 90 degree angle from your torso.

Keep your arms straight at your sides, palms up.

Contract your abdominal muscles, elongate your neck and press your lower back into the mat. **[1**

FORM CHECK:

■ Bring your legs closer to your body if the exercise becomes too difficult.

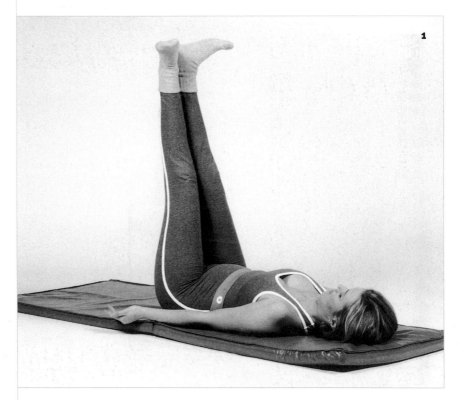

1

advanced mermaid

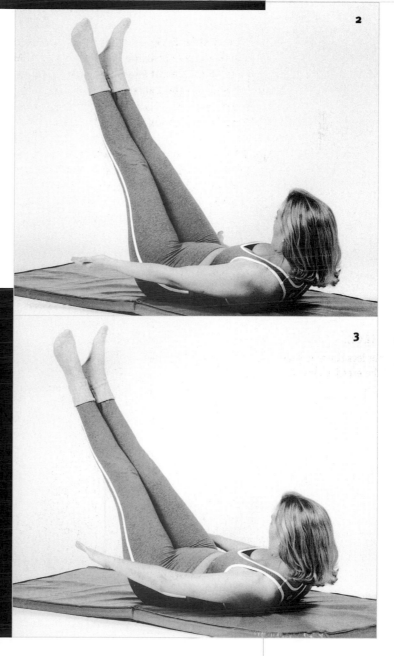

2

3

THE MOVEMENT

- Lift your shoulders and upper back off the mat as high as you can go as you lower your legs about a third of the way down from the angle at which you started. Raise your arms to the height of your hips.

- Pulse your arms, palms up, for the count of six, breathing in. [2

- Pulse your arms, palms down, for the count of six, breathing out. [3

- Repeat six times.

- Leaving your legs in the starting position, lower your upper body to the mat.

- Bend your knees and lower your legs.

exercise **eight**

THE PURPOSE   After all your intense effort, you deserve a break. As your breath fills your lower, then mid- and upper back, feel how your rib cage relaxes.

START   Lie on your stomach with your arms at your sides. Turn your head to the right side and rest it there.

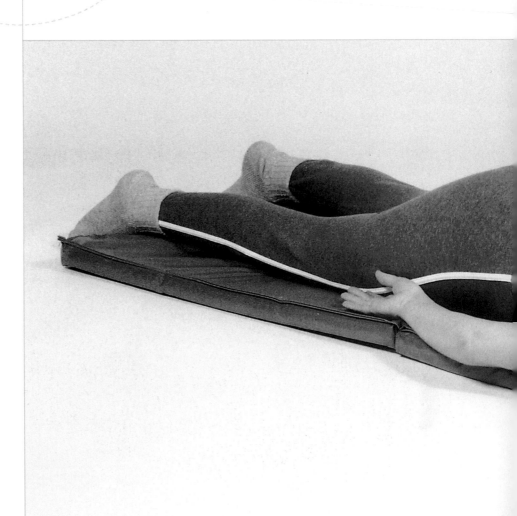

belly breath

THE MOVEMENT

- Take a long, slow breath through your nostrils, filling up your lungs as you silently count to four.
- Hold the breath for seven seconds.
- Exhale through your nose as you count out loud to eight.
- Turn your head to the left side and repeat.

TIPS:

- As you inhale, imagine the warm air flowing to all parts of your body.
- As you gently exhale, imagine the tension flowing out of all your muscles.

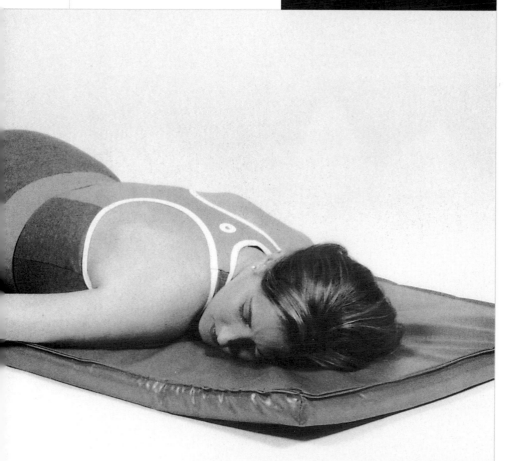

exercise **nine**

THE PURPOSE This powerful intensifier of the Core Foundation movement involves ankle weights and hand weights. Begin by using one-pound ankle and hand weights for three weeks, then try to increase to two-pound ankle and hand weights for the next three weeks. After that, see if you can increase to three-pound hand and ankle weights—your Ultimate goal.

With so many muscles now strengthened and your posture dramatically improved, standing and sitting taller will be easier than ever.

START Put on your ankle weights.
Lie on your stomach with your forehead resting on the mat.
Holding a one-pound weight in each hand, extend both arms straight out in front of your head. Elongate the back of your neck, tighten your abdominals and press your pubic bone into the mat. **[1**

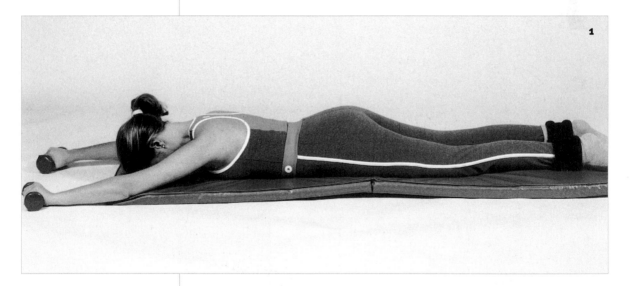

1

FORM CHECK:

- Keep your head facing down, and the back of your neck long and straight.

- Be sure to keep your pubic bone pressed into the mat for spinal stability.

super cross extension

THE MOVEMENT

- Extend your right arm in front of you as far as possible and lift it three to six inches while simultaneously raising your left leg three to six inches with the toes pointed. **[2**

- Hold the position as you count out loud for six seconds, and then release.

- Return to the starting position and repeat with the opposite arm and leg. **[3**

- Repeat three times.

TIP:

- Think of reaching forward with your hand and backward with your foot as far as you can.

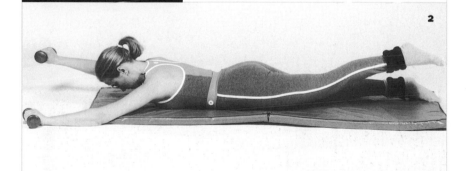

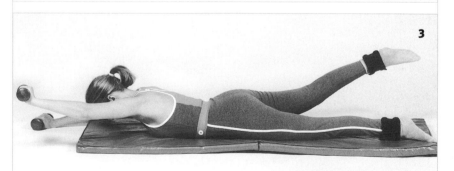

NOTE: *Remove your ankle weights in preparation for the next exercise.*

exercise **ten**

THE PURPOSE   This is such a superlative exercise that I've included it one more time. After the effort of working with weights, it provides you with a well-deserved full-body extension.

START   Lie on your stomach with your chin just above the mat. Place your palms on the mat, at the sides of your shoulders. Keep the tops of your feet resting on the mat. [1

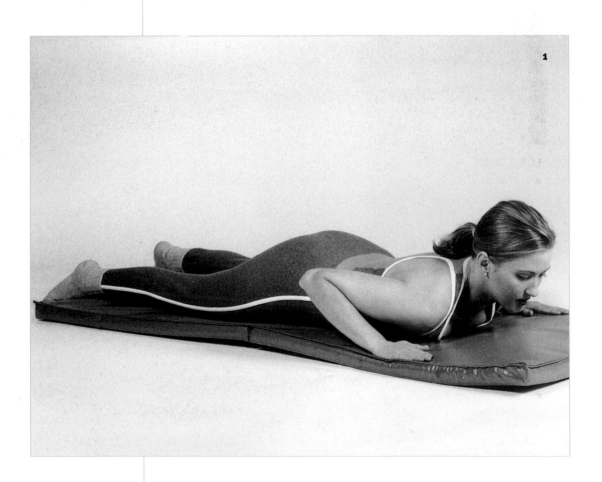

1

the cobra

THE MOVEMENT

- Push up, tilting your head back slightly, in the sequence of forehead, nose and chin. **[2**

- Face forward as you rise, pushing up on your arms and opening your chest, keeping your pubic bone pushed into the mat while relaxing the buttocks as best you can.

- Slowly arch your spine backward, straightening, but not locking, your elbows.

- Roll your head back and look up at the ceiling. **[3**

- Hold the position as you count out loud to three and then descend slowly to the mat.

- Repeat six times.

FORM CHECK:

- As you begin your stretch, imagine your spine as a banana that you are slowly peeling from your neck, mid-back, then lower back.

- Instead of tightening your buttocks as you lift off the mat, which limits the spinal extension, just press up with your arms into the range that is most comfortable. With each repetition, attempt to press up higher, keeping your buttocks relaxed.

- Keep your back relaxed and "flaccid." Don't hunch your shoulders together. Let your arms do the work — great for triceps toning.

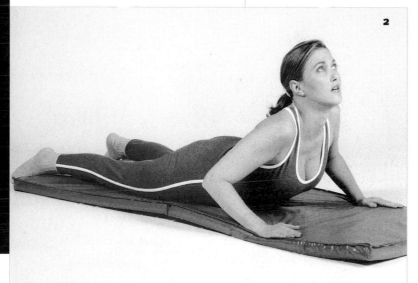

2

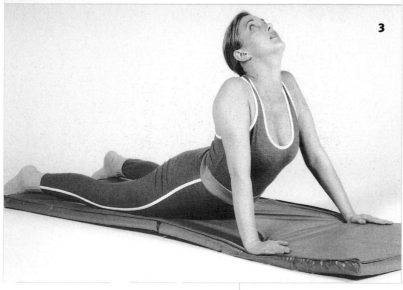

3

exercise **eleven**

There is no better way to finish a workout than to let all of your muscles relax. Do it exactly as you did before.

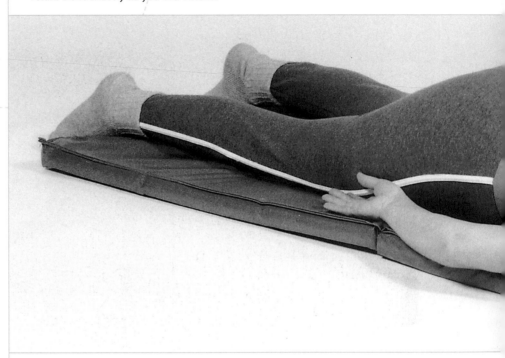

POWERFUL TO THE CORE!

You have just completed the Ultimate Core. This means that you are doing all that you can for your body. It will function and feel and look great today and for the rest of your life!

I want to remind you that you can switch back and forth between the Core Programs depending on how you are feeling. All will give you benefits. There may be times when you feel the Ultimate Core is too strenuous. Maybe you had the flu for a week. Perhaps, like me, you recently had a baby. As soon as I was able, I went back to the Core Foundation while continuing to do the Sun Salutation from the Ultimate Core. I found that any minor hot spot discomforts I was feeling soon disappeared, and I was able to work my way back to the Ultimate Core very quickly.

belly breath finale

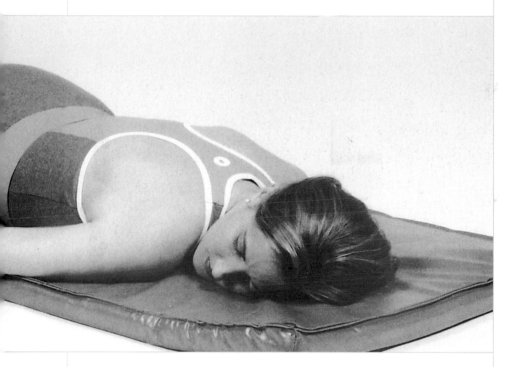

GOOD FOR YOU!

You're stronger and straighter than ever before, and you are looking—and feeling—younger.

I know from my patients that their motivation keeps increasing the more they do the Core Programs. This is because they know that if they don't do the Programs, they will soon begin to feel stiff and achy. They won't move as comfortably or stand as straight. And that is no longer acceptable to them, because they've had the experience of feeling good all the time.

I know you'll have the same reaction. Why would you accept feeling any less than great, right down to the core?

1. Sun Salutation

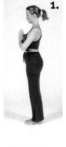
1.

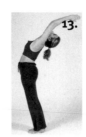
13.

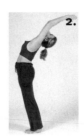
2.

3.
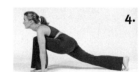
4.

5.

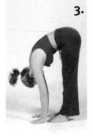
12.

6.

11.
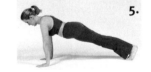

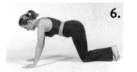
10.

9.
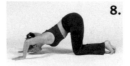
7.

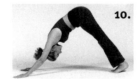

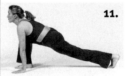

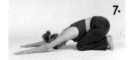
8.

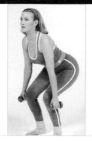

2. Squats

3. Double Dead Bugs

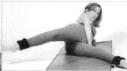 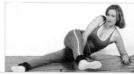

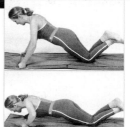

4. Push-Ups

5. Butterfly with Weights/Heel Beats with Weights

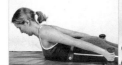 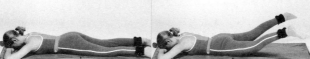

6. Three-Part Advanced Pelvic Stabilizer

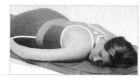

7. Advanced Mermaid

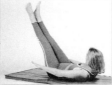

8. Belly Breath

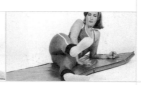

9. Super Cross Extension

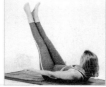 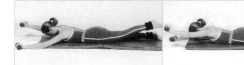

10. The Cobra

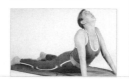

11. Belly Breath Finale

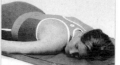

Keeping Fit to the Core

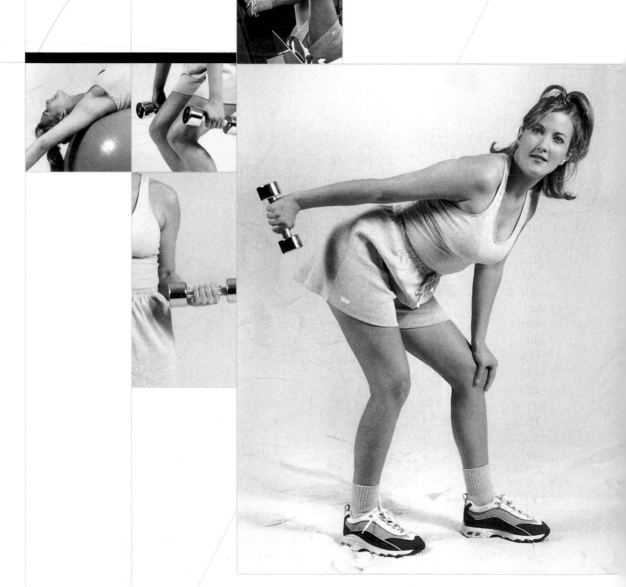

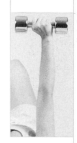

weight training: the ideal complement to the core program

EVERY WOMAN CAN BENEFIT FROM WEIGHT TRAINING

It's very important to remember that, as a woman, you will gradually lose 1 percent of your muscle mass every year after age 40—unless you do resistance training. Not only will this make you weaker, but it will make you fatter too, because less muscle tissue means you burn fewer calories.

I regard resistance, also known as resistive, or weight, training as an important part of a woman's fitness strategy. Weight training, whether it's done with machines, or with dumbbells and ankle weights, builds muscle and bone mass, and enhances strength, balance, circulation, mood and metabolism. At the same time it reshapes bodies by reducing body fat, cuts the risk of osteoporosis, diabetes and heart disease, increases endurance and bolsters self-confidence. As you can see from the photos in this chapter—taken when I was three months pregnant—I continued my weight-training during my pregnancy, to help keep me strong for everything I would need to do after the birth of this second child.

The whole idea of resistance training is based on the overload principle. For instance, if you expect a muscle to be able to lift five pounds, when you exercise you lift seven pounds. This ensures that you will always be able to lift five pounds.

BEFORE YOU BEGIN

Whether you already use weight-training equipment, or are just getting started, the first thing you should know is that the equipment you find in gyms, and the exercises taught in most books and by most trainers, were developed by men, for men, based on men's upper-body strength and lower-body structure. The second thing to know is that there is a right way and a wrong way to use resistance equipment. With the best intentions, many fitness experts and personal trainers perpetuate less-than-ideal ways to use resistance equipment because they don't take into consideration the strain on a woman's joints, much less her body alignment and muscle balance. In the exercises that follow, I've given information about proper form, and, as I did in the Core Programs, I've included a number of Don'ts to enable you to correct some common mistakes in workout form. I've also told you about a number of exercises to avoid altogether. Though they are part of many basic training regimens, they can easily lead to injury.

MAKE THE MOST OF YOUR WORKOUT

Here's some basic information you need about how to combine the Core Program with weight training, and how to make your workouts as effective—and injury-free—as they should be.

- Add your resistance workouts to the days you do the Core Program.
- Divide your resistance workouts, concentrating on the upper body two days a week, allowing at least a day between workouts, and then working the lower body two other days, again with at least a day between workouts. The reason for allowing time off between workouts of the same sets of muscles is simple. When you build muscle it needs some recovery time. A sample workout schedule might look like this: Work your upper body on Sunday or Monday and Wednesday, and your lower body on Tuesday and Friday or Saturday.
- If you do weight resistance on a day you aren't doing the Core Program, warm up with the Sun Salutation (page 178) before you begin, to assure flexibility.
- A workout should take you about fifteen minutes.
- Do one set of each exercise, with twenty-five repetitions. This will give you toned muscles and a time-efficient workout.
- Do each exercise this way: The muscle contracting (concentric) phase is done for the count of two. The muscle holding (isometric) stage is done for the count of one. The muscle elongating (eccentric) phase is done to the count of four. The slower release gives you maximal toning effect.
- When lifting weights, avoid locking joints at the end ranges of the movements, in order to protect yourself against tendinitis and joint strain.
- You can determine when it's time to add weight this way: If you can do the release phase of the last five reps to the count of six, then it's time to add another plate to your resistance equipment or increase the weight of your dumbbells.

- Do a Sun Salutation as a cooldown.
- The exercises are presented in the order that they should be performed. They recruit the muscles of the torso first, and then work the muscles of the extremities. Information on which muscles are being worked, and why, is included. The first round of exercises described below works the upper body; the second round works the lower body.

DO AN AEROBIC WARM-UP

I strongly advocate aerobic training for women. With heart disease the number one cause of death in American women, I feel it's imperative that women do aerobic exercise, which offers a terrific cardiovascular workout. I recommend doing twenty to thirty minutes of aerobics three times a week, as a complement to the Core Program. Your aim is to work up to your Target Heart Rate, which is 70 to 80 percent of a figure arrived at by subtracting your age from 220. For a 40-year-old woman, the Target Heart Rate, or number of heartbeats per minute, would be somewhere in the range of 70 to 80 percent of 180, or 126 to 144. Once you've warmed up, the target rate should be sustained for the duration of your aerobic workout.

If you are doing resistance training, starting with a 15-minute aerobic workout will give your heart health a boost and also warm you up for the exercise to follow. You can cross-train if you wish—that is, do five minutes on each of a choice of several aerobic machines. I recommend using a stationary bicycle. My favorites for comfort are the semi-recumbent cycles, such as the Cybex or the Lifecycle. Another machine that gives you a good cardiovascular workout is the NordicTrack, which I like because it engages your stomach muscles—without your having to think about it—while you move your arms and legs. Two other excellent machines are the Stepmill, revolving stairs which provide perhaps the most challenging cardiovascular workout, and the UBE, or Upper Body Ergonometer, which you work by pedaling your arms in a cycling motion, from a position in which they are elevated above your heart. If you use the UBE, go backward instead of forward most of the time. This will pull you up and out rather than down and in. And finally there's the StairMaster. If you use it for your cardiovascular workout, be sure to follow the directions on page 228 in order to avoid the strains that commonly result from poor posture while on this machine.

The injury-free resistance workout: upper body

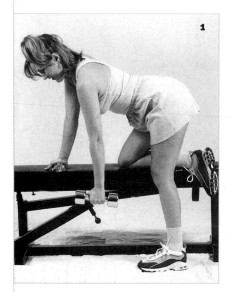

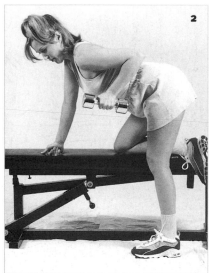

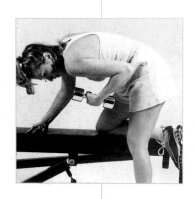

These first two exercises work the middle trapezius and rhomboid muscles. By bringing the shoulder blades closer to the spine, these exercises increase stability and build arm power.

Bent-over Row on Bench:

- Place one leg on the floor with the other knee on the bench. [1
- Pull your shoulder blade toward your spine as you pull your elbow alongside your torso and lift the weight. [2

Bent-over Row on Bench:
DON'T

Don't round your back or bend your wrist. You'll use your biceps but you won't isolate the middle back muscles, which is the aim of the exercise.

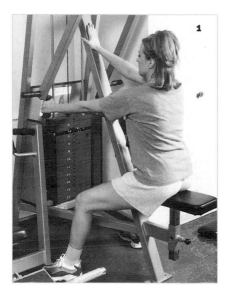

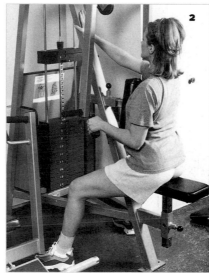

One-Arm Row on Row Machine:

- Sit straight up on the machine and grasp the vertical handle. **[1**
- Pull the handle back toward your body as you lift your chest. **[2**
- Pull your shoulder blades down and in toward your spine.
- Release slowly.

One-Arm Row on Row Machine:

DON'T

Don't round your back. The middle back muscles won't be isolated as intended, and you might pinch the nerves exiting from the bottom of the neck.

Two-Arm Row on Row Machine:

AVOID

Don't work both arms at the same time. Doing so will create too much joint compression in your upper back. Also, it won't isolate the muscles you're trying to work.

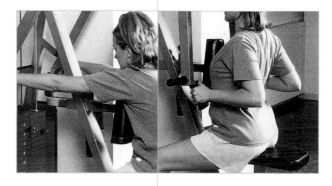

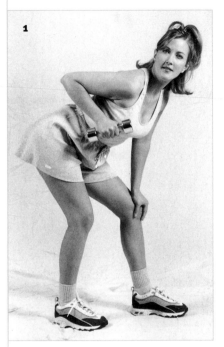

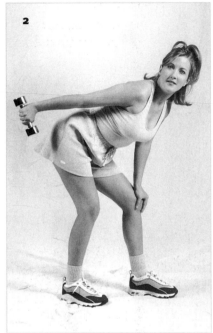

These next exercises work the triceps, toning the muscles under and in back of the arms.

Triceps Kickbacks:

- Bend knees in a lunge position with a straight back; bend at the hips. Place the hand without a weight on the front of your thigh for support.
- With bent elbow, lift weight to chest level. **[1**
- Extend arm backward with straight wrist. **[2**

Bench Skull Crushers with Weights:

- Lie down on the bench with knees bent. Bend your arms to a 90 degree angle, letting the weight clear the top of your head. **[1**
- Straighten your arms and bend them in a controlled, slow manner. **[2**

Bench Skull Crushers with Weights:

DON'T
Don't extend your arms too far over your head. Although you'll be working the triceps, you may injure the soft tissues of the shoulder joint. Also, don't lock your elbows when your arms are straight.

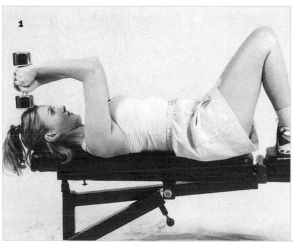

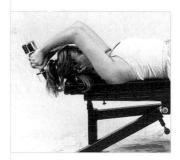

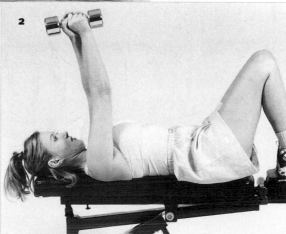

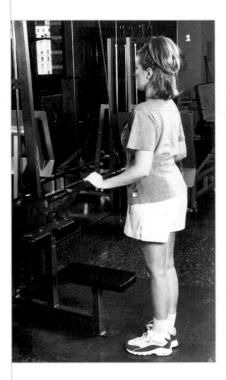 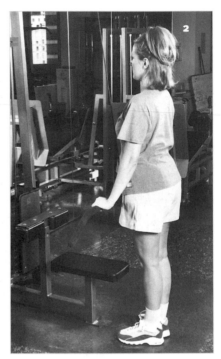

Triceps Press-Downs:

- Grasp the latissimus bar with a shoulder-wide grip, and keeping your arms against the sides of your torso, pull the bar down until your elbows are bent at a 90 degree angle. **[1**
- Straighten elbows without locking them, pushing the bar down against the resistance of weights, and then bring your elbows back to the 90 degree angle. **[2**

Triceps Press-Downs:

DON'T

Don't lock the elbow when it's extended. You want to avoid joint compression and tendinitis.

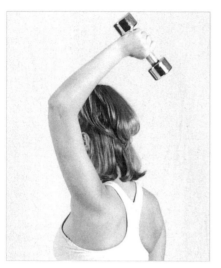

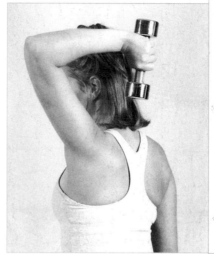

Overhead Triceps:
AVOID
Don't do this free-weight exercise in which you move a weight up and down in back of your head. This can cause shoulder impingement and joint dysfunction.

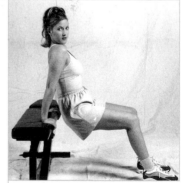

Triceps Bench Dips:
AVOID
Don't lean back on the bench and press up and down as shown. If you do, you can create shoulder strains and spurs.

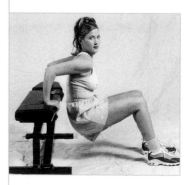

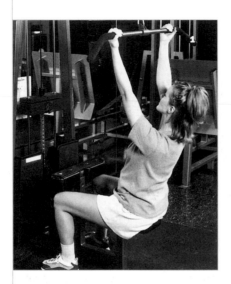

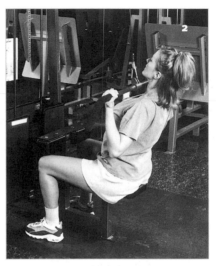

The following exercise works the latissimus dorsi, which pulls the shoulder blade down and back. The result gives your waistline a V look.

Front Lat Pull-Downs:

- Sit on the machine, leaning back, and hold the bar with your palms facing you. **[1**
- Pull the bar down to chest level in front of your face as you lift your chest. **[2**

Front Lat Pull-Downs:
DON'T

Don't pull the bar down behind your head. The forward head posture promotes stress and strain on the nerves, joints and muscles of the lower neck. Furthermore, this improper movement will only encourage poor posture.

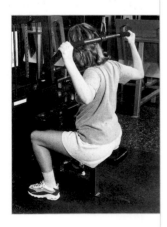

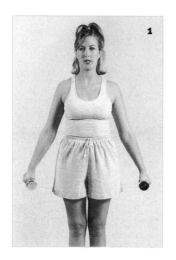
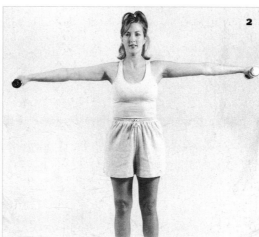

The next exercise works the deltoids and rotator cuff muscles. Doing so tones the shoulder muscles and stabilizes the shoulder joints.

Lateral Raise:

- Hold dumbbells down and out at your sides. [1
- Extend both arms sideways to a 90 degree angle. [2
- Slowly lower them with your chest lifted and shoulders back. This will give you proper postural alignment.

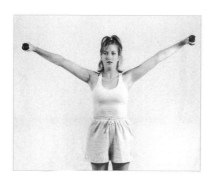

Lateral Raise:

DON'T

Don't lift dumbbells too high. Raising arms above the horizontal will impinge on the rotator cuff tendons and create an inflammation that will give you bursitis or tendinitis.

Overhead Press with Dumbbell:

AVOID

Because of the excessive compression forces on shoulder joints, this exercise can cause shoulder impingement, bursitis and tendinitis.

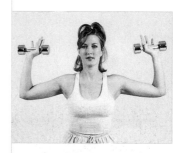

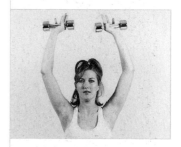

The next exercise tones the pectoral muscles, which will firm your chest and lift your breasts.

Bench Chest Press with Weights:

- Lie on your back with bent elbows and knees, holding the dumbbells so that your upper arms are parallel to the floor. [1

- Press the dumbbells up toward the ceiling, straightening your arms to almost their full extension. [2

- Flex your arms back to the starting position. Doing the Chest Press in this midrange recruits the most muscle fibers and generates optimal strengthening.

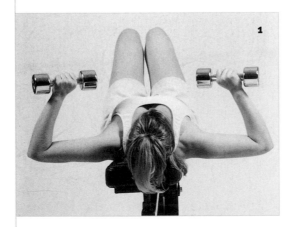

Bench Chest Press with Elbows Dipping:

DON'T

Don't let the elbows drop below chest level. If you do, a strain will be placed on the front of the shoulder joints.

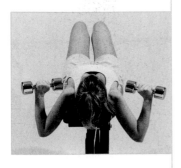

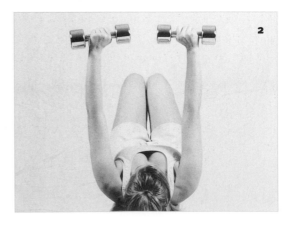

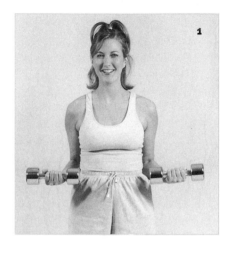
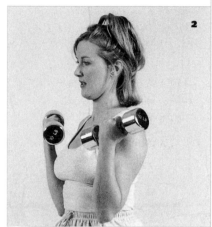

The following exercise works the biceps muscles and strengthens the arms, which makes carrying things much easier.

Biceps Curls:

Pull in your abdominal muscles to stabilize your spine. This will prevent your back from arching.

- Hold weights at waist level. **[1**
- Lift your chest and pinch your shoulder blades together.
- Curl the weights to your shoulders. **[2**
- Slowly lower the weights until your elbows are fully extended.
- Release the contraction slowly to maximize the recruitment of biceps muscles fibers and avoid excessive elbow compression.

Biceps Curls:

DON'T
Don't lean back. If you do, you'll lessen the effectiveness of the exercise and put unnecessary strain on your back.

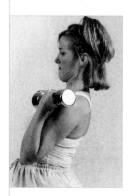

The injury-free resistance workout: lower body

The first exercise works the calf muscles and tones them while strengthening ankles.

Heel Raises:

There are two variations, the first with straight legs, the second with bent knees. Before both, tighten your inner thighs by imagining that you're holding a volleyball between your knees. The purpose is to keep your ankles from rolling outward.

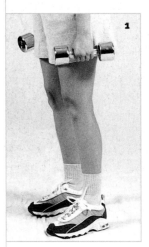 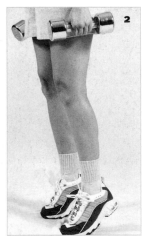

Straight Leg Heel Raise

- Stand, with hands at sides, holding dumb-bells. [1
- Go up on your toes keeping your knees straight. Go down and up with straight legs 25 times. [2

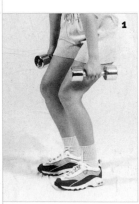 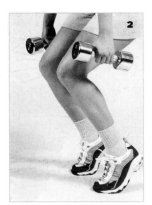

Heel Raises:

DON'T

Don't let your ankles roll outward. Instead of strengthening calf muscles to prevent ankle sprains, you will contribute to possible injury by twisting the ankle joints and overstretching your ankle ligaments.

Bent Knee Heel Raise

- Bend your knees. [1
- Go up on your toes with your knees bent. Keeping knees bent, lower and raise your heels twenty-five times. [2

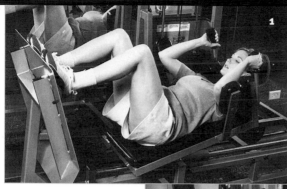

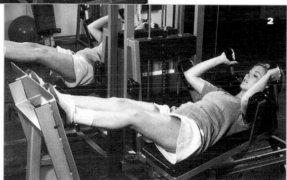

Note: You can also do a one-leg version of this exercise. When doing one leg at a time, let the unengaged leg hang down, with knee bent, off the panel. Working one leg at a time will create even more power in each leg, and give you more control when you walk up and down steps. **[3, [4**

The next exercise strengthens all the lower-leg muscles, especially the hamstrings and quadriceps, giving you added power when you are walking, running or playing sports.

Leg Press:

- Lying down with your lower back pressed firmly against the carriage, bend your knees 90 degrees and place your feet on the panel. Hold the handrails. **[1**
- Press your feet flat against the panel and push away from it until your legs are almost straight, stopping before your knees lock. **[2**

Leg Press:

DON'T

Don't lock your knees when you straighten them. Doing so strains the knee joints and inhibits maximal recruitment of all the quadriceps muscles.

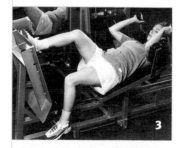

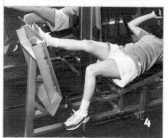

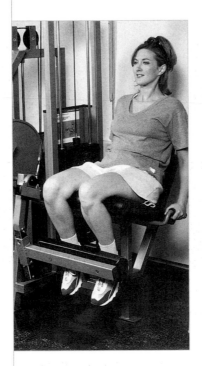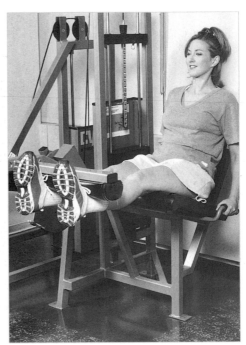

Knee Extension Machine:

AVOID

Using this machine compresses the kneecap into the femur, thereby increasing the stress on the knee and promoting premature degeneration behind the kneecaps. If you do this exercise, you may start feeling pain in the knees when walking down stairs, which is the first symptom of chondromalacia, a common knee problem.

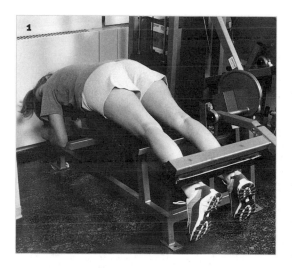

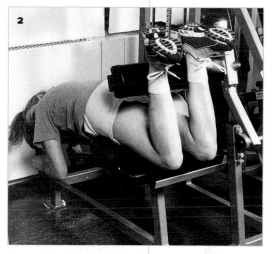

The following exercise works the hamstring muscles, which gives you stronger legs and prevents your knees from hyperextending.

Hamstring Curl:

Tighten your stomach to keep your spine aligned. Keep your spine in neutral position, not arched or rounded.

- Lie facedown on the bench, with your knee joints aligned with the axis of the curling bar and with your ankles underneath the pads, so the pads rest just above your heels. Hold the handles on either side of the bench. [1

- Bend your knees and slowly lift the bar all the way up so the pads touch your buttocks. [2

- Slowly lower the bar.

Hamstring Curl:

DON'T

Don't let your buttocks rise when you pull the bar up. Decrease the weight if you find you cannot keep your buttocks from rising.

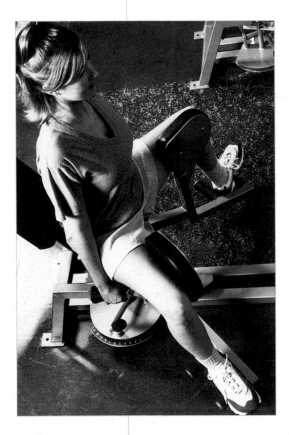
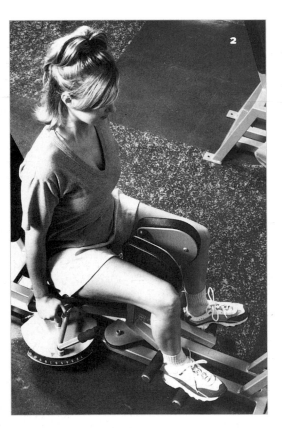

The next exercise works the adductor muscles, which tone and strengthen the inner thighs.

Hip Adductors:

- Sit on the machine with your legs apart; place your hands on the handles by your hips. [**1**
- Pull your legs together, keeping your spine straight, and slowly release them. [**2**

The next exercise works the abductor muscles, which strengthen and tone the outer thighs. It also works the gluteus medius, which gives proper hip and knee alignment.

Hip Abductors:

- Sit up straight on the machine (not leaning back) with your legs together; place your hands on the handles. **[1**
- Push your legs apart, and slowly release them. **[2**

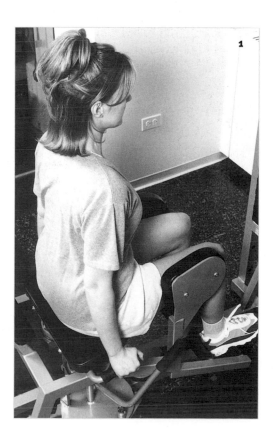
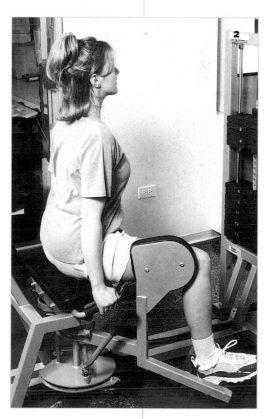

The following aerobic exercise helps to tone the lower body.

StairMaster:

Stand erect, as you stair-step, holding your head straight up, and keeping your hands on the bar.

StairMaster:

DON'T

Don't rest your arms on the bar and bend over with your head facing down. This position strains the lower back and puts excessive shearing forces on your sacroiliac joint (where the pelvis meets the spine). Weakness, as well as dysfunction while walking, can result.

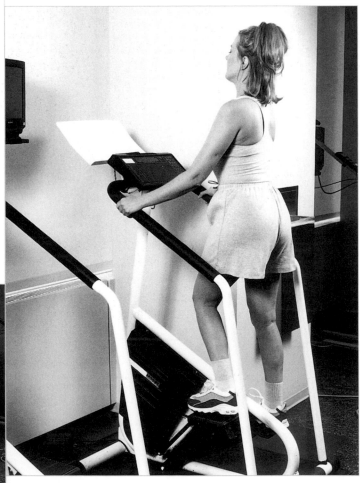

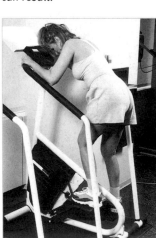

winding-down exercises

After my workout, here are two exercises that I like to do.

Ball Stretch.

If your gym has a large rubber ball, like the one pictured here, take advantage of it. Arching backward over the ball, with your arms extended over your head, will give you a terrific pectoral stretch that expands your chest, as well as all the muscles of respiration.

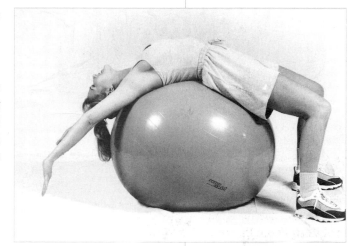

Wall Postural Isometric (bonus exercise).

Performing the following movement will strengthen your transverse abdominis.

START

Stand with your back against a wall with your pelvis tilted. Your heels, about six inches apart, should be one foot length away from the wall, legs straight or slightly bent. Place your arms at your sides, palms forward. Keeping your lower back close to the wall, lift your chest and bring your shoulders back against the wall, too. Now tuck in your chin to elongate your neck and bring the back of your head in contact with the wall as well.

THE MOVEMENT

- Pull up and in with the muscles of your abdomen to flatten your midback against the wall. Hold this position for about six seconds.
- Relax.
- Take a deep breath, inhale and exhale.
- Repeat six times.

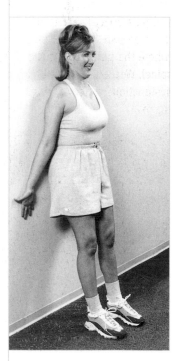

IF YOU FEEL SORE AFTER A WORKOUT

For relief of muscle soreness, there are several things you can do:

- Think cold. Cold acts as an analgesic, or pain reliever, as well as an anti-inflammatory. If, however, you can't tolerate cold, alternate it with heat, which will relieve muscle spasms. Then apply cold once more. Use a package of frozen peas or corn kernels, placed inside a pillowcase to protect your skin from frostbite. Apply the cold pack to the sore area for ten to twenty minutes. Don't let your skin turn red; if this happens it means that cold has been applied too long.

- Remain active if possible. After two or three days, even if you're still sore, a very light repetition of the same, or similar, activity that brought on the soreness will help loosen your muscles and decrease the inflammation without further injuring the muscles.

- Take aspirin or other anti-inflammatories only as necessary for a short period (two to three days). If you are taking other medications, consult your physician. If you can't tolerate aspirin, use acetaminophen as a pain reliever.

YOUR LIFESTYLE CHECKLIST

Keeping your body healthy can be summed up easily. Ideally, you will do:

- the Core Program
- resistance training
- aerobic conditioning

You will also need:

- enough sleep (eight hours a night)
- at least eight eight-ounce glasses of water a day
- something or someone to bring you joy each day
- food that is highly nutritious

Nourishment is very important. In order to keep your furnace stoked and your energy levels constant throughout your busy day, you must choose foods that will deliver a nutritional boost. Doing so will not only make you feel better—you'll be getting the energy you need to resist gravity for efficient posture.

I give my patients some basic nutritional guidelines because food is the first line of defense for achieving and keeping a healthy body. It can also help offset signs of premature aging.

First of all, you need protein—like fish, lean meat, poultry and eggs—because it supplies eight essential amino acids the human body does not manufacture itself. Four ounces of protein three times a day will supply your body with these essential building blocks, which build muscle. Omega-3 fatty acids, found in flaxseed and salmon, are excellent for nourishing joints. They also prevent

You Are What You Drink

More than anything else, our bodies consist of one thing: water. Water makes up 85 percent of blood and 75 percent of the brain. Muscles, which are 70 percent water, must be kept hydrated. Muscle dehydration of just 3 percent leads to a 10 percent reduction in the strength to contract and an 8 percent reduction of speed.

The conductor for all the electrical impulses and chemical reactions that constantly take place, water also lubricates joints.

So drink up. Eight to ten eight-ounce glasses of water daily (and more if you drink coffee or alcohol, which are dehydrating) will give your body the fluid it needs to function smoothly.

When You Should Stop Exercising

Stop your workout immediately if you experience any of the following:

- Difficulty breathing
- Chest pain
- Dizziness or a feeling that the room is spinning
- Extreme pain
- Feeling uncomfortably hot
- Nausea
- Numbness or loss of sensation in any body part
- Throbbing headache
- Fever

Consult your physician before beginning another workout.

blood clots and artery-clogging plaque, which are factors in heart disease. Studies suggest that the oils in fatty fish also offer some protection against osteoarthritis.

Second, nine servings of fruits and vegetables a day provide nutrient-dense fuel—and they count as carbohydrates. A serving size is easy: It's just a fistful. Many dark leafy green vegetables contain calcium, which can help ward off osteoporosis. Of course that's only one of dozens of health benefits you get from fruits and vegetables.

WHAT WORKS FOR ME

This is the eating plan I follow because it keeps me feeling satisfied while giving me the fuel I need to get through my day without crashing.

Breakfast: I like to eat three different fruits and then have eggs. The fat in the eggs keeps me satisfied and maintains steady blood sugar levels. And the fruit, full of nutrients, contains lots of fiber, which stimulates bowel elimination.

Lunch: I have a salad and vegetables along with whatever protein I choose.

Snack: I always keep a four-ounce bag of low-fat pretzels with me. (I keep a cannister of pretzels in the waiting room of Brill Physical Therapy.) Munching on these prevents a drop in my blood sugar levels.

Dinner: If I decide to have pasta I cook three fistfuls of pasta and add three fistfuls of vegetables. It's hearty and delicious and comforting.

I save weekends for what I like to call my discretionary food fund. That's when I'll indulge in dessert or whatever else I feel like.

Read Labels and Protect Your Joints

Many processed foods, especially baked goods, contain partially hydrogenated oils. Research suggests that these substances make the bloodstream acidic, which, in turn, creates acidosis in joints. The result wears down cartilage, which can lead to osteoarthritis.

Stop the Three O'Clock Slump

If you want to eradicate the three o'clock letdown, don't eat starchy grain carbohydrates (like pasta or bread) along with protein for lunch. Doing so will set up a competition between the two for enzymes in your digestive tract. Your pancreas will produce extra insulin to absorb the sugar, which is a by-product of starchy carbohydrate digestion. Your blood sugar will spike up and down, leading you to crave a boost—like more sugar, or caffeine from chocolate or coffee. Your body will have to work harder to metabolize your food and you will feel tired.

Liniments

Many people rub liniments on sore muscles. These liniments, most of which contain camphor, oil of turpentine or oil of wintergreen, create a feeling of warmth by dilating blood vessels on the surface of the skin. Although safe when used as directed by the label's instructions, liniments have only a superficial effect. Unable to penetrate deeply enough through either the skin or the fat layer above the muscles to reduce soreness, liniments don't promote healing. What these ointments and gels may do, however, is temporarily block pain signals to the brain. Also, the self-massage stimulates circulation and may bring temporary relief from the soreness. Liniments won't hurt you—but don't expect too much from them, either.

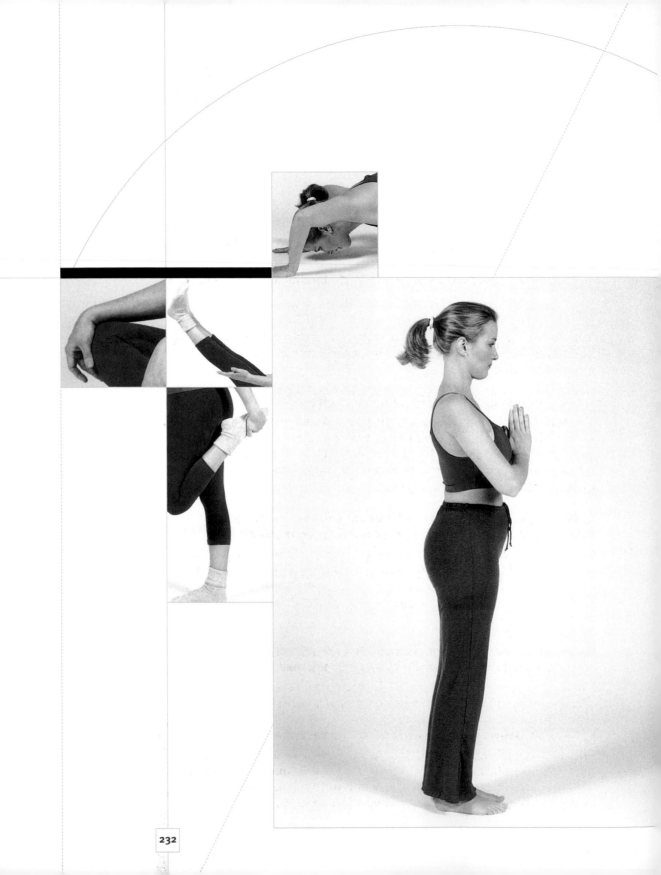

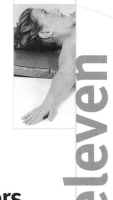

questions and answers

The Core Program has generated many interesting questions from my female patients. Here are some of the most frequently asked questions, and my answers.

Q. Will I lose weight doing the Core Program?

You will lose inches and tone your body. As far as losing pounds goes, doing the Core Program will augment any weight-loss program you are on, especially if you also do aerobic exercise and resistance training. Proper diet should be part of any healthy regimen—including the Core Program.

Q. My six-year-old daughter watches me do the exercises and then mimics me. Is she too young to do the movements?

Good for her! No, she isn't too young—and I believe it's never too early to instill the habit of regular exercise in children. Look at the extra benefits you're both receiving: You're exercising at home so the two of you are spending time together, and you're having fun. What could be better?

Q. Every month I suffer from excruciating menstrual cramps. Should I skip doing the Core Program on those really bad days?

No, and for a very good reason: The movements enhance overall circulation, which will help relieve some of your discomfort.

Q. Can I eat before I perform the Core Program?

Since the exercises involve the stomach muscles, eating too much food too close to exercise time can lead to uncomfortable gastric distress. If you eat a big meal, allow one to two hours before exercising to give yourself adequate digestion time. If, however, you feel the need to eat something before your workout, try a banana, an apple or yogurt. These foods tend to digest easily and settle comfortably in the stomach.

Q. I have scoliosis. Can I do the Core Program?

Yes, you can. The exercises help to restore skeletal balance, which is what you need to do. The core exercises are prescribed for many of my scoliosis patients.

Q. I'm trying to become pregnant. Is it okay for me to do these exercises?

Of course. The Core Program should be part of an all-around good-health prepregnancy regimen since it builds your strength and stamina. It prepares abdominal and pelvic floor muscles to support the weight of the growing baby throughout pregnancy.

Q. A couple of years ago, I discovered that I have a mitral valve prolapse. Is it okay for me to do the Core Program?

Absolutely. The exercises help pump blood to all the body's muscles, including the heart, and improve circulation throughout your extremities.

Q. I had a mastectomy last year. Is it safe for me to perform the core exercises? What benefits will I receive?

The Core Program is definitely safe to do once you have healed from surgery. You will notice improved circulation, decreased swelling throughout your arms, improved posture and a reduction of incisional adhesions along your chest wall. The exercises will also help prevent frozen shoulder, which is commonly seen in postmastectomy patients.

Q. I understand that my entire body will be getting lots of terrific benefits from the Core Program, but I have to ask: Will any of the exercises actually flatten my stomach?

Yes. Perform the Dead Bugs and Mermaid in the Intermediate or Ultimate Core regularly and you'll see your belly start to decrease in size. These exercises recruit all the abdominal muscles, strengthening while elongating them in the process.

Q. While we're at it, will any of the exercises help me get rid of the "saddlebags" I carry on my thighs?

It's a legitimate question, especially since you will be working your legs and buttocks so thoroughly. You'll be glad to know that several of the exercises, particularly the Three-Part Pelvic Stabilizer in the Core Foundation, will help reduce "saddlebags" by improving muscle tone in your thighs. The addition of ankle weights in both the

Intermediate and Ultimate Core Programs makes this exercise even more effective.

Q. Do the facial exercises really work?

Yes, they do. To prove it to yourself, take a "before" picture and begin the exercises. Three weeks later take an "after" picture and then compare the two photos. You be the judge.

Q. I like the idea of progressing from one program to the next, but I don't think I can lift the weights in the Intermediate Core. What should I do?

First, start without weights. After you get comfortable with the exercises, add the lightest weights, increasing them by a pound every two weeks, until you finally reach the desired weight.

Q. I just had knee replacement surgery. Will the Core Program work for me?

It certainly will. The Core Program will help stabilize your hips and pelvis, which will give you increased knee stability.

Q. I've suffered for years with chronic arthritis. Is the Core Program safe for me to perform?

Let me reassure you. The core exercises won't hurt you, whether you have osteoarthritis or rheumatoid arthritis. In fact, they will help you prevent joint imbalances and, therefore, further wear and tear on your joints. Another benefit is temporary pain relief, because the stress on the joints will be relieved. However, you are the best judge of what works for you, so let any discomfort be your guide. If you feel uncomfortable doing any exercise, cut the number of reps in half, or divide the Core Program into two segments. Do half the exercises in the morning, and the rest later in the day, until you can comfortably tolerate doing the entire program in one block of time.

Q. Although I'm still active, I'm hesitant to try the Core Program because of a recent diagnosis of multiple sclerosis. What do you recommend?

The Core Program has helped patients of mine with MS to increase their balance, stability and strength. The exercises are challenging enough to provide muscle strengthening yet not so vigorous that they become debilitating.

Q. I have an embarrassing problem. I get awful foot cramps whenever I'm stuck in a long meeting. Since it would be awkward to get up and walk around the conference room to ease them, is there anything else I can do to make those cramps go away?

You need to stretch your calves—a lot. When you do the Progressive Hamstring Stretch, do three times the number of reps prescribed for the third and fourth parts—the Ankle Pump and Steel Thighs. Doing so should correct the muscular imbalance and relieve those annoying cramps.

Q. For years, my husband has complained about my cold feet. Short of wearing socks year-round, is there something I can do to warm them up?

Yes, there is. Cold feet—and hands too—are often caused by improper breathing. If you don't exhale thoroughly, you won't rid your body of excess carbon dioxide. Too much carbon dioxide in the blood causes vasoconstriction of blood vessels and, consequently, cold extremities. The remedy is deep breathing. See pages 85–86 and follow the easy directions.

Q. Because of my queasy stomach, I pop a lot of antacids. Is there any other way to ease my discomfort?

You'll be happy to know that you can stretch your way to better digestion. The Core Program includes movements that stretch the soft tissues around the nerves that feed into the stomach. Doing these movements will inhibit the activity of the nerves, which results in a "calmer" stomach. (A proper diet helps, too. See the reading list for guidance on nutrition.)

Q. I want the Core Program to be as effective as possible. What can I do?

Maximizing the benefits is easy. Just follow the basic "rules of wellness." Drink eight to ten glasses of water, and eat nine servings of fruits and vegetables, plus three four-ounce servings of lean protein every day. Get eight hours of sleep a night, nourish your joints by eating fish several times a week, breathe properly and think positive thoughts about all the good things you're doing for yourself. And keep your body moving! Once you've seen the results, share the Core Program with someone whose health you care about.

A Final Word

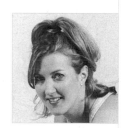

It "drives me crazy" whenever I hear anyone who has simply resigned herself to poor health, whether on account of illness or injury, or as part of the inevitable process of aging. If you empower yourself with the knowledge to make wise choices about how you live, then there is nothing inevitable about pain and dysfunction. That is why I urge all of my patients to educate themselves about their bodies, to take advantage of the unprecedented wealth of information now available to help them maintain lifelong health and wellbeing.

Exercise is the number-one antidote to aging. If you have embarked on the Core Program exercises, congratulations! You are on the way to becoming balanced and strong. That means you will sit, stand and move in the ways nature intended, secure in the knowledge that your body will be able to face whatever challenges it meets, confident that it will be able to do whatever you want it to. Every day you will wake up refreshed and invigorated, free of discomfort and pain.

So please let the healing effects of exercise enter your life. Exercise your right to feel fabulous—and you will, today and every day, right down to the very core of your being!

Good health consists of more than just having a physically fit body. There are many other factors involved in becoming truly healthy that fall outside my own field of expertise. But as someone who wishes to empower her patients to make wise choices based on an understanding of all the ways they can be proactive in pursuit of good health, I often recommend books on a variety of topics, including diet, intimate relationships, positive feelings and attitudes, spiritual path, stress management, sense of purpose and meditation. The journey to health—physical, emotional, mental and spiritual—is a lifelong path involving discovery and self-renewal. May these books inspire you as they did me and give you hope for ever-greater health and happiness in the future.

Please use selections from this list of my favorites to help you become an effective advocate for your own health. The experts who wrote these books will be good companions on your journey, giving you knowledge and insight that will light the way.

Eight Weeks to Optimal Health
by Andrew Weil, M.D.

Cliff Sheats' Lean Bodies
by Cliff Sheats and Maggie Greenwood-Robinson

Your Personality, Your Health
by Carol Ritberger, Ph.D.

Getting the Love You Want
by Harville Hendrix, Ph.D.

recommended reading

You Can Heal Your Life
by Louise L. Hay

Prescription for Nutritional Healing, 2nd edition
by James F. Balch, M.D., and
Phyllis A. Balch, CNC

The Change Before the Change
by Laura E. Corio, M.D.

Women's Bodies, Women's Wisdom
by Christiane Northrup, M.D.

The Wisdom of Menopause
by Christiane Northrup, M.D.

index